HOMEGROWN
CANNABIS

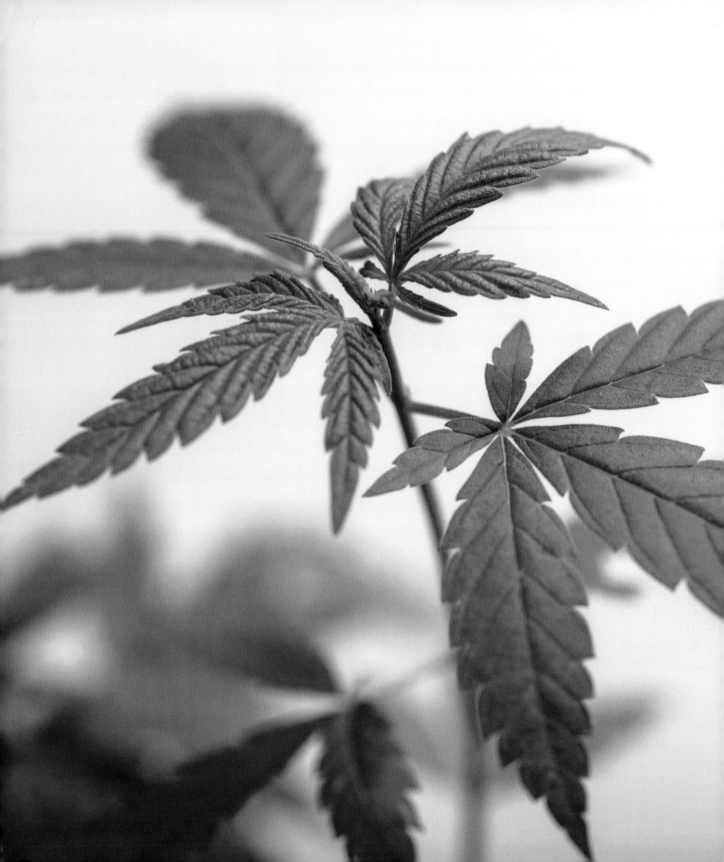

HOMEGROWN CANNABIS

A BEGINNER'S GUIDE TO CULTIVATING ORGANIC CANNABIS

Alexis Burnett

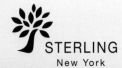

STERLING
New York

STERLING
New York

An Imprint of Sterling Publishing Co., Inc.

ISBN 978-1-4549-4209-2
978-1-4549-4210-8 (e-book)

Distributed in Canada by Sterling Publishing Co., Inc.
c/o Canadian Manda Group, 664 Annette Street
Toronto, Ontario M6S 2C8, Canada
Distributed in the United Kingdom by GMC Distribution Services
Castle Place, 166 High Street, Lewes, East Sussex BN7 1XU, England
Distributed in Australia by NewSouth Books
University of New South Wales, Sydney, NSW 2052, Australia

For information about custom editions, special sales, and premium and corporate purchases, please contact Sterling Special Sales at 800-805-5489 or specialsales@sterlingpublishing.com.

Manufactured in Spain

2 4 6 8 10 9 7 5 3 1

sterlingpublishing.com

Cover design Jo Obarowski and Igor Satanovsky
Interior design by Gavin Motnyk and Shannon Nicole Plunkett
Picture credits—see page 236

CONTENTS

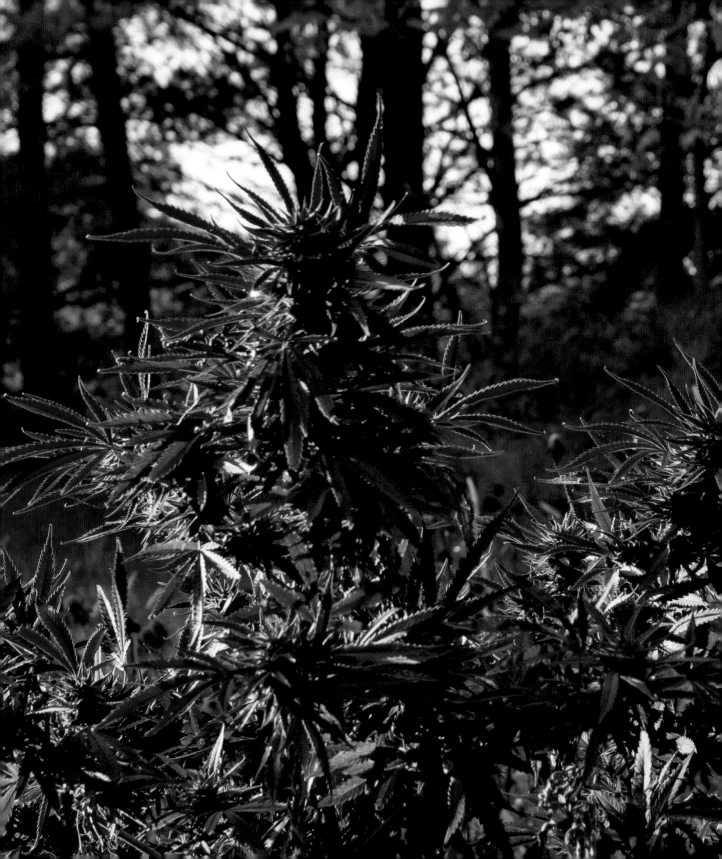

< INTRODUCTION >

Cannabis is one of the oldest known cultivated plants. Physical evidence of its use dates back approximately twelve thousand years. Cannabis is thought to have originated in central Asia, and humans have brought it to places around the world. It has worked its way into many different cultures and the lives of many people, used for everything from food, medicine, and building materials to spiritual rituals. For most of its history with humans, this plant has been revered, respected, and used without stigmas, skepticism, and stereotypes. In the last hundred years, however, things began to change. We moved into the dark days of prohibition, and this plant, at least in the West, and the people who used and relied on it had to go underground.

As we move into the world of legalization, we enter a time where many are being reintroduced to cannabis. As the laws change from state to state and country to country (with Canada being just the second country, after Uruguay, to fully legalize cannabis), more people can grow and use this plant without fear of being prosecuted.

When I was first introduced to cannabis cultivation, this plant instantly enthralled and enchanted me. I knew right away that I would work with cannabis for many years to come. I've grown cannabis every season since that initial interaction, both indoors and outdoors. Through these growing seasons, I have seen it help hundreds of people. Although it was illegal to grow it at the time, I was willing to take this risk in order to better understand this master plant and all that it has to offer. I was interested in how to grow cannabis in a way that showcased its medicinal qualities, produced the cleanest medicine, and left the soil, the earth, and all of nature stronger and more vital as a result. There were many successes as well as many failures. I absorbed important lessons over all of these years. My understanding of this plant and how to cultivate it to its optimum potential has grown with each passing season. The times are changing, and as I reflect on the many experiences of the past, I also look forward to a brighter future where more people can grow and work with the cannabis plant.

LEFT One advantage of growing cannabis at home is the ability to select cultivars (see page 9) that best suit your needs. Pictured here is a Glazed Cherries plant glistening in the setting sun.

I am proud that my hands can nurture this healing plant to produce bountiful, cannabinoid- and terpene-rich flowers that can change the lives of those they touch. I've had a passion for sharing my experiences growing this plant with others for many years, and with cannabis now legal in Canada, I have begun to teach a number of courses on growing, medicine making, and the history of this fascinating plant, both online and in person. I've outlined much of the information in this book and hope that you will take this knowledge and share it far and wide as we all learn to grow, care for, and work with this important healing plant.

REASONS TO GROW CANNABIS

Why grow cannabis? Well, if it is now legal to cultivate this plant where you live, why not? By growing cannabis yourself, you can be sure that your plant has been grown without the use of pesticides or chemical fertilizers. It will also save you money. Buying cannabis from a dispensary or another government-regulated store can be expensive, but it can be grown outdoors, under the sun, using organic and regenerative principles (see page ix), harvested at the optimal time, and cured to perfection for just pennies a gram. Plus, cannabis is such a stunning and spectacular plant that it will add grace and beauty to any garden.

With laws on using and cultivating cannabis changing, there has never been a better time to learn to grow this plant at home and in your backyard gardens, especially if you are a medical cannabis user. If you grow cannabis at home, you can choose the cultivars that best suit your condition and produce the effect that you are looking for. Your homegrown cannabis has the potential to be far superior to anything you could buy, and you can be sure that it has been grown with love and care and in a way that is respectful and in balance with the natural world.

So, grow your own cannabis, be proud, and take your health and enjoyment into your own hands. Your experiences with homegrown cannabis will allow you to develop a relationship with this plant, one that will last a lifetime. And you will enjoy the feeling of empowerment that comes with a successful harvest.

HOW TO USE THIS BOOK

This book is for the beginner to intermediate grower and has been written with a focus on organic and regenerative growing practices. I have designed this book to guide you through the growing process from seed to harvest and to show you how you can grow your own top-quality cannabis at home step-by-step.

Although I will cover the basics of setting up an indoor growing space and share tips for indoor growing throughout the book, this book will focus mostly on growing your plants outdoors under the sun—what we in the cannabis community affectionately call sun-grown. I will show you ways to grow cannabis outdoors, whether you live in an apartment building in a major city and grow your plants in pots on your balcony or in a rural environment with space for large beds. I have outlined a strategy to achieve results that you can be proud of and supply you with clean, organic cannabis.

Each chapter builds on the previous one and guides you along through each of the growing stages as your plant matures. I recommend that you follow the processes in the order outlined until you have at least one successful harvest under your belt. After you have gained more experience and understand this plant on a deeper level and in a more intimate way, you can begin experimenting with different growing styles and techniques and even create approaches that fit your unique environment, needs, and goals. There is no one right way to grow this plant, but it is important to start with the basics and build a solid foundation on which you can "grow" your experience.

WHAT IS REGENERATIVE FARMING?

Regenerative farming was designed as an alternative to conventional farming and consists of practices and techniques that help to rejuvenate the soil and the environment. These practices include avoiding soil tilling, sequestering carbon in the soil, using natural organic inputs to support the growth of your plants, and eliminating reliance on synthetic fertilizers and chemical pesticides. While regenerative farming techniques can be considered sustainable or environmentally friendly, they go beyond simply maintaining existing systems and conditions by giving us ways to make the world a better and healthier place. Regenerative farming is about building resilient systems that give back to the land and its many inhabitants. It offers ways to work with your native soil and increase the beneficial fungal and microbial life that resides there, making them readily available to your plants. These living soil systems, along with the energy of the sun, create healthy plants and support almost all life on earth.

We can apply regenerative farming techniques to growing cannabis in our home gardens. By doing so, we not only increase the health and vitality of our plants but also help our farms, backyards, homes, and communities thrive. I believe that gardening is a remnant of our role as caretakers of the earth, one that our ancestors played for thousands of years. Through observing nature and thinking about the life and health of the soil, environment, and community from a regenerative standpoint, we can continue playing this role by bringing balance and harmony back into the spaces and land that we steward, no matter how large or small that area may be.

Growing plants in soil using organic growing methods and principles is an important part of regenerative farming. The methods include designing and utilizing holistic systems that strengthen the diverse communities of life on our farms, backyards, and world, from the microscopic life in the soil to the bees, butterflies, birds, and mammals with which we share space. Using these principles means striving to create, maintain, and expand biodiversity in whatever space you work with. For example, by using nutrients from organic or living sources (such as manure and compost), we avoid relying on synthetic fertilizers, chemical salts, and harmful chemical pesticides. These nutrients tend to be more ecologically sustainable and are released slowly, which decreases the possibility of overfertilizing and potentially "burning" your plants.

Regenerative cannabis farming goes beyond simply using organic practices by integrating closed-loop systems into your garden or farm. By using closed-loop systems, you can limit the number of inputs that need to be purchased from outside sources and brought to your property, often by finding ways to use by-products or "waste" that you may generate. For example, a farm creates a closed-loop system when it raises animals, such as chickens, and uses their excrement as fertilizer for its plants and gardens. Repurposing this by-product from the animals adds nutrients and beneficial organisms to your soil, which in turn feeds the plants, thus eliminating the need to bring in store-bought fertilizers or other off-site nutrients. This also allows us to use resources that would have been used to manufacture, package, and transport those off-site products for other purposes. Through these practices and others like it, you are giving back to the land and not only *sustaining* the vitality of your ecosystem but also *regenerating* its health and productivity.

Each element or component in your garden or on your farm can perform many functions. These are what we call "stacking functions." In the example above, chickens offer many stacking functions. You can harvest eggs and meat from the chickens. Those chickens provide manure for the garden, help till and scratch up new garden beds, provide a source for feather and bone meal, and eat insects—the list goes on and on. Stacking functions can offer additional ways to close other loops in your systems.

Another important principle of regenerative agriculture is understanding the myriad of ways that everything in the natural world is connected. It is important to learn to view your garden, no matter how big or small it is, as part of the bigger system. We do this by observing how our garden affects all the life that surrounds and lives within it. For instance, growing plants such as cannabis naturally, outdoors and under the sun, gives us a chance to see how they fit into the bigger picture, allowing us to observe both the plants and the natural systems around them. The more time we spend in nature and outside with our plants, the more we can learn about the natural world and our place within it. You may find yourself surprised at how much you are learning about your environment solely by growing, taking care of, and spending time in your cannabis garden.

Because your garden is part of a larger system, the choices that you make impact your environment and your community. If you want to practice regenerative principles and methods, you need to take these impacts into account. Always consider whether your actions are restoring or bringing health and vitality back to the land. If not, look for ways that you can bring balance back to the natural rhythms of the earth. As you plan your garden and begin growing cannabis, ask yourself these questions: Are your choices positively affecting all the plants, animals, and people with whom you share your space? How was a product manufactured, and where was it harvested or mined from? How far did it travel to get to your store? What was the economic and environmental cost to get a product, input, or nutrient? In supporting a product, are you making the world a better place for future generations?

When we begin to look at our cannabis-growing inputs (and all the choices we make in life) through this lens, we can begin to make a serious and lasting change in the way that we interact with the earth. Regenerative farming and cannabis growing comprise a journey. As you practice regenerative growing techniques with cannabis, you will need to get to know your garden, property, and ultimately bioregion on an intimate level—this is not something that can be done in a short period of time. This process can take years, and it grows and evolves with the grower and their relationships to the plants, land, and community. It depends on forming relationships, sourcing local inputs, cultivating an awareness of your impact on the place you live, and looking to nature for the support, inspiration, and lessons in resiliency that can be applied to other aspects of your daily life. It involves enhancing and creating biodiversity in your gardens and on your land.

There is no doubt in my mind that the regenerative techniques outlined in this book will benefit you by producing the cleanest, best-tasting, low-impact cannabis possible. I hope they will also benefit the earth and future generations. As the cannabis industry expands and big business interests enter this grassroots community, it is more important than ever to learn, grow, and show people that there are ways to work with this plant that bring us back into balance with the environment, ourselves, and our communities.

Practicing regenerative agriculture techniques as craft and small-scale home growers can set an example for others to follow. By practicing these principles, we can begin to give back. And by giving back, we begin to make the world around us a better place to live for us and all life. The smallest of actions can build over time and have a great and lasting impact. If you are going to grow cannabis, why not make choices that have a smaller footprint on the environment and support health and biodiversity in the ecosystem?

COMMON REGENERATIVE FARMING PRACTICES

Although it may appear that you need to have land or a farm to implement regenerative farming practices, this is not true. No matter where you live, there are many things that you can do at home, in a city or a small town, that fit the bill. Every action that you take can have a positive impact, and if we all do our part, we can make a tremendous change in the health of our planet. Here are some examples of common regenerative farming practices to try at home.

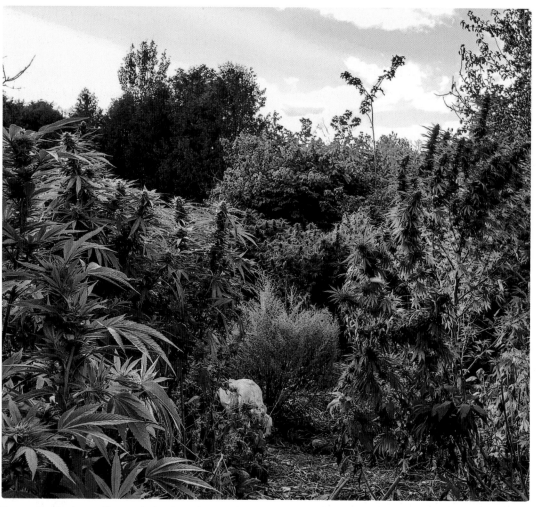

Regenerative farming practices can be done in any home garden, no matter its size. For example, companion planting—which creates a polyculture garden where many different plants, shrubs, and trees grow together in one environment—can be implemented on a large scale, as shown here, or in a container garden.

- Create a compost pile or bin, or vermicompost—compost made with the help of earthworms. Gather leaves from neighborhood trees for mulch and compost.

- Reuse and build soil. Discarding old potting soil is not a sustainable practice when it can be reused and reamended for future growing seasons.

- Save seeds (and breed your own cannabis seeds). Gathering and saving seeds makes you less dependent on outside sources. In the old days, there were very few seed banks, and the ones that did exist did not make seeds readily available for purchase. It was up to the farmer to save seeds for future crops.

- Grow your own food and other medicinal herbs. There are thousands of medicinal plants you can grow besides cannabis. Supplying yourself and your family with your own source of food and medicine allows you to take your health and nutrition into your own hands and avoid depending on anyone else to supply your needs.

- Plant polyculture gardens. By planting a polyculture garden, you can see and experience firsthand the positive impact that growing different types of plants can have on your environment. Growing cover crops (see page 192) and practicing companion planting techniques (see page 45) can help your garden and your local ecosystem thrive. For example, vegetables or culinary and medicinal herbs will benefit not only you but also the many insects that will pollinate, feed, and take shelter in these diverse plantings.

- Make locally harvested inputs and fertilizers, such as compost and fermented plant teas (see page 132), to limit your use of store-bought pesticides and nutrients.

- Encourage biodiversity. Plant flowers and pollinator gardens to attract beneficial insects to your garden.

- Build rainwater catchment systems. Water is a resource that is not plentiful in all parts of the world. Gathering rainwater will ease the pressure on our groundwater systems and conserve valuable drinking water.

- Practice no-till techniques (see page 45), and utilize mulch (see page 103) and cover crops (see page 192) to protect bare soil. Repetitively tilling soil is harmful to the microbial and fungal life that resides there. These organisms are important, as they help our plants to absorb important nutrients needed for growth.

- Build community and share resources. Educate others about regenerative farming.

Cannabineae.

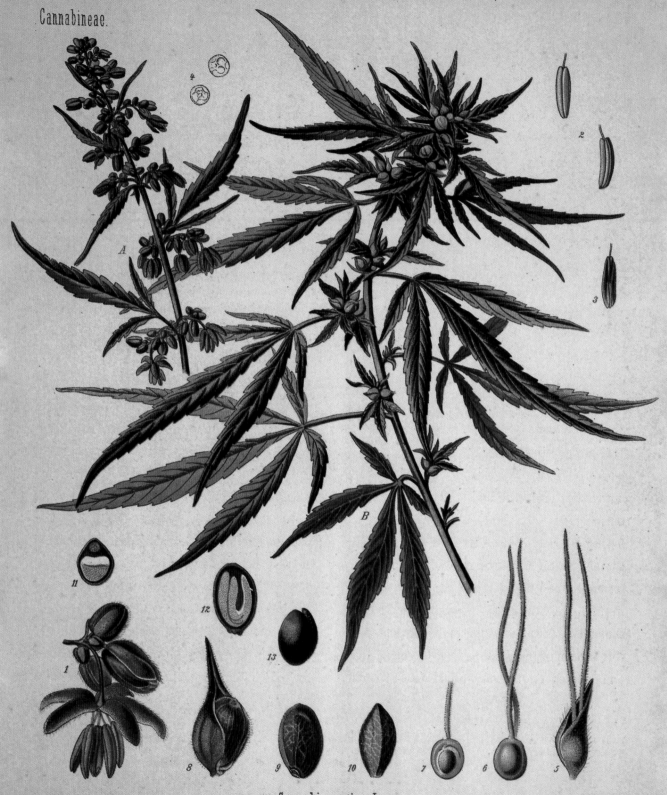

Cannabis sativa L.

W. Müller.

CHAPTER 1

< Cannabis Botany >

Botanists, researchers, and laypeople know and agree on many things when it comes to the cannabis plant, such as its physical structure and its chemical constituents. But when it comes to areas like its taxonomic classification, there is more disagreement. This chapter will convey what is considered common knowledge in the cannabis community and industry, and some ideas that may be considered controversial when it comes to classifying cannabis and explaining how it affects us when we use it. Understanding the botany and classification of cannabis will add another level to your knowledge base as a grower. When you combine this information with personal growing experience, you will be well on your way to forming a well-rounded and deep relationship with this plant.

The prohibition against cannabis has made it hard for universities to study this plant without the fear of losing licenses and facing criminal charges. Fortunately, as cannabis becomes legalized or decriminalized in many countries throughout the world, there is now more money, resources, and bright minds studying the plant in intense detail. As more information becomes available to the public, some of the information in this section of the book may need to be changed and updated. For anyone who has studied plants before, you are most likely aware of the fact that botanists are constantly changing the classifications of many plants as more genetic data and research information becomes available. That said, the information found in this chapter should be more than enough to get you started and, if this subject is of interest, you can go down the botanical and classification rabbit hole as far as your heart desires. I have mentioned my sources for information that I provide in this chapter for you to follow up on and research on your own.

LEFT This nineteenth-century botanical drawing shows the parts of a male *Cannabis sativa* plant, one of the three species of cannabis. While you may see different varieties of cannabis described as "indica" or "sativa," there is debate among scientists and growers about whether this distinction is the best way to classify them.

< 1 >

THE PARTS OF THE CANNABIS PLANT

Cannabis is a flowering plant that stands upright, has branching leaf veins, and produces seeds from a flower. It is a dioecious plant, meaning there are male and female flowers on separate plants. When most people think about cannabis, they think of the female flowers or buds, as they are commonly called. It is the female plants and flowers that are most commonly grown and used, but some growers use the male plants for breeding.

CANNABIS PLANT ANATOMY

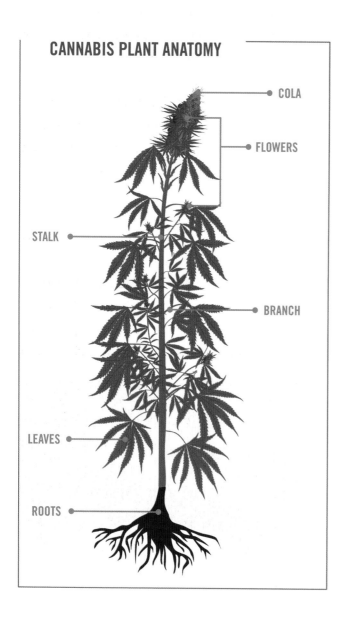

- COLA
- FLOWERS
- STALK
- BRANCH
- LEAVES
- ROOTS

BOTANICAL NOMENCLATURE OF CANNABIS

Kingdom: Plantae (Plants)

Subkingdom: Tracheobionta (vascular plants)

Superdivision: Spermatophyta (seed plants)

Division: Magnoliophyta (flowering plants)

Class: Magnoliopsida (dicotyledons)

Subclass: Hamamelididae

Order: Rosales

Family: Cannabaceae

Genus: *Cannabis*

Species: *Cannabis sativa, Cannabis indica, Cannabis ruderalis*

Roots

The cannabis plant has a taproot that grows deep into the earth and many fine, fibrous secondary rootlets. The roots of the cannabis plant anchor it into the ground and draw up nutrients from the soil that move upward through the central stalk.

Stalks and Branches

The central stalk of the cannabis plant grows rapidly toward sunlight. The side branches push out from what is called a node. Nodes are generally arranged in pairs on the central stalk in an opposite branching pattern, though individual nodes may appear near the top of the plant in an alternate branching pattern. The space between the nodes is called internodal spacing. Generally speaking, cannabis plants that evolved closer to the equator in warmer climates have larger internodal spacing, meaning that they have fewer branches. Plants that evolved in colder climates have tighter internodal spacing, meaning that they have densely arranged branches.

Leaves

The leaves of cannabis are perhaps the best-known part of the plant. The iconic image of cannabis leaves has been associated with the plant and the culture (and counterculture) of cannabis enthusiasts the world over. The leaves are generally arranged across from each other on opposite sides of the stem, but on some plants individual leaves alternate sides. The same plant may display both opposite and alternate leaf arrangement. The cannabis plant has palmately compound leaves that resemble the shape of a hand. Each leaf consists of five to nine leaflets.

The leaves capture sunlight for photosynthesis, producing food for the plant from the energy of the sun. They are full of vitamins, minerals, and flavonoids. Many people will juice them or add them to smoothies.

There are smaller and often single-blade leaves that are located close to the flowers or intermingle with them. These leaves, often called sugar leaves, are covered in trichomes and can be used when making your own cannabis products.

Trichomes

Trichomes are resin glands that are largely concentrated on the flowers, though they will be found in lower concentrations on the stalk, some leaves, and the male flowers. They are very sticky and give the cannabis flowers a shiny, glistening appearance. The trichomes contain and secrete a

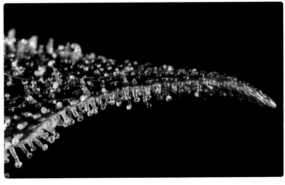

Capitate-stalked trichomes (*shown here*) produce and contain many of the cannabinoids and terpenes found in cannabis.

resinous substance that consists of terpenes (see page 108) and various cannabinoids. It is these trichomes that carry the main medicinal and psychoactive constituents of the cannabis plant, and they are highly sought after. There are three types of glandular trichomes:

- **Bulbous trichomes** are the smallest type. These glands are located on the surface of the entire plant. They are 25–30 microns in height with a 20-micron diameter head.

- **Capitate sessile trichomes** are larger and more abundant than bulbous trichomes. The heads measure 40–60 microns in diameter and are flush with the surface of the plant.

- **Capitate-stalked trichomes** are slightly larger still and contain both a head and a stalk. The head of these glands can measure up to 100 microns. These are the most bountiful and abundant of the three trichomes and can be easily seen with the naked eye. The glandular head of each trichome serves as the center of terpene and cannabinoid production.

All these trichomes produce cannabinoids, but the capitate-stalked trichomes are most abundant in and around the calyxes of budding flowers (also known as sepals). They produce the highest concentration of essential oils, due to their size.

In addition to containing the cannabinoids, flavonoids, and terpenes, trichomes act as a deterrent to animals and insects that may want to feed on the plant. They protect the plant from UV rays and from drying out by reducing the amount of air that circulates around the plant.

Flowers

Cannabis flowers form on both the male and female plants. The male plants will have male staminate flowers, and the female plants will have female pistillate flowers. In the odd case, some plants will become hermaphroditic, meaning there will be both male and female flowers on the same plant. Hermaphroditic plants often have a few flowers of the opposite sex that are scattered on a branch or two, rather than appearing throughout the whole plant.

Both male and female plants will show signs of pre-flowers at around 6 weeks of age, sometimes later. These pre-flowers, also known as primordial flowers, are the earliest signs of the plant's sex. The male pre-flowers will have a small round, "ball-like" structure, and the female pre-flowers will show one or two pistils or hairs protruding from a small calyx.

The male flower buds have five radial segments that form inside a calyx. A calyx, consisting of the sepals, protects the flower as it develops. The calyx opens up to a flower with five petals that are about 5 millimeters long each and vary in color from white to green or yellow. Each flower

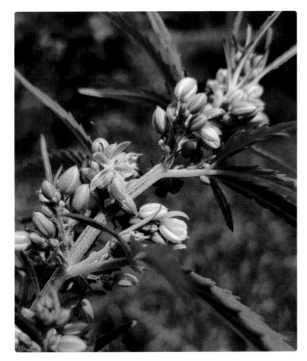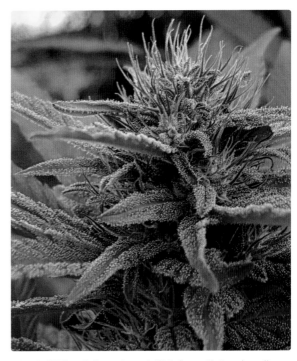

LEFT Male flowers have staminate flowers with "sacs" that produce and release pollen. RIGHT Female flowers have pistillate flowers that receive pollen from male flowers to form seeds. The pink hair-like tendrils shown in this photo are the flowers' pistils.

has five 5-millimeter stamens consisting of pollen sacs known as anthers, which are attached to a thin filament. Male plants tend to grow quicker and taller, and they flower a little earlier than female plants. Male flowers develop in clusters, and after opening, they will drop yellow, dust-like pollen. The plants tend to die back shortly after dropping pollen.

Female flowers have two hairlike pistils that extend from a thin, light green calyx that is covered in trichomes. The calyxes are between 2–6 millimeters in length and contain a tubular ovary. When fully mature, the pistils will be about ¼- to ½-inch (6–13 mm) long. Once the flower is pollinated, the pistils die back, and a seed begins to form in the ovary. Seeds take between 4 and 6 weeks to form, and have spotted or striped black, brown, and gray patterns. The female flowers are generally the most sought-after part of the plant. Flowers that are not pollinated are called sinsemilla (from the Spanish phrase *sin semilla*, which means "without seeds"). Sinsemilla flowers will continue to grow bigger as they anticipate the arrival of pollen for reproduction.

Most cannabis is photoperiod-dependent, meaning the plants begin to flower as the days get shorter during the end of summer and early fall.

Autoflower cultivars will begin to flower after a specific period of time has passed (usually within 3–4 weeks), regardless of the amount of daylight that they receive.

A grouping of calyxes from a female plant form what is called an inflorescence. The longer apical or terminal buds are referred to as the "cola"; the cola is the set of elongated spikes on the top of a flowering female cannabis plant. When covered in trichomes, colas will have a frosty appearance and give off a strong and beautiful scent.

HERMAPHRODITE FLOWERS

Hermaphrodite plants contain both male and female flowers. Oftentimes, these plants will not show these traits until later in the flowering stage. Plants will develop hermaphroditic traits because of poor genetics or improper breeding practices. Environmental stress from fluctuating temperatures, chemicals, light leaks, interrupted light cycles, and nutrient deficiencies can also cause a plant to grow both male and female flowers as well.

The male flowers on hermaphrodite plants will pollinate the female flowers in your garden, passing this undesirable genetic tendency toward hermaphroditism down to their offspring. It is best to get rid of hermaphrodite plants quickly before they become a problem. You do not want to have these plants pollinate others in your garden and spoil your entire crop.

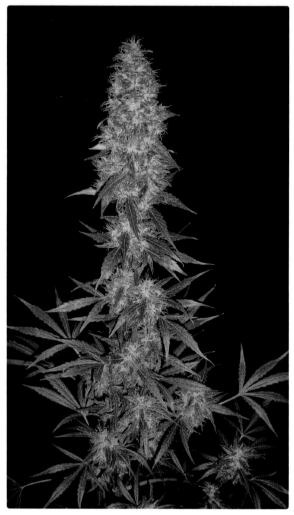

A cola can contain hundreds of flowers and can grow more than 2 feet (60 cm) tall and more than 6 inches (15 cm) wide.

CLASSIFYING CANNABIS

Cannabis species have been classified in many different ways over the years. In 1753, Carolus Linnaeus proposed that cannabis was monotypic, consisting of only one species, called *Cannabis sativa*. In 1785, French biologist Jean-Baptiste Lamarck distinguished between two species: *Cannabis sativa*, a taller more fibrous plant, and *Cannabis indica*, a shorter more psychoactive plant. For two centuries, this polytypic thinking prevailed before the majority of botanists reverted to a monotypic classification of one species again—*Cannabis sativa*. In the 1970s, a number of scientists and scholars, including Dr. Richard Schultes, an ethnobotanist at Harvard University, proposed that the genus *Cannabis* includes three distinct species: *Cannabis sativa*, *Cannabis indica*, and *Cannabis ruderalis*.

The earliest botanists, such as Carolus Linnaeus, used morphological differences to describe and ultimately classify different cannabis species, rather than focusing on the effects of smoking or ingesting these plants. This way of classifying cannabis, which is still used today, is often misleading and does not correspond well to the way that cannabis interacts with our endocannabinoid system and makes us feel. Laws have also played a big part in how cannabis has been and will be classified around the world. (It is much easier to outlaw one species of plant than two, three, or more.) To make things more complicated, cannabis has traveled the world and been bred by humans, who have selected for different traits at different times in history.

Many people in the cannabis industry often associate certain effects of cannabis with specific species. It is assumed that sativa plants will induce an energetic and uplifting effect, while indica plants will induce a sedative or "couch-lock" effect. This is simply not true. There has been so much hybridization between these species that there are very few plants that we would call "pure" sativas or indicas. In addition, it is the presence of various cannabinoids and terpenes, and the ways these compounds interact with your body, that produce specific effects, not the way the plant looks. In recent years, there have been studies that have looked at cannabis cultivars at a genetic and chemical level in hopes of better understanding their differences on a molecular level.

In their comprehensive text *Cannabis: Evolution and Ethnobotany*, Robert C. Clarke and Mark D. Merlin, drawing from the work of biologist Karl Hillig, then proposed a new way to classify cannabis, based on an approach that combines morphology and its effects on the body. It is this system of classification that we will talk about here. It challenges some commonly held beliefs about how cannabis is described in today's current climate, but it also provides some much-needed distinction between the various subspecies of cannabis in a way that is easy to understand. As we learn more about cannabis, there will inevitably be changes in the coming years to how cannabis is classified.

There are two categories of cannabis: hemp varietals, which are used as food, fuel, and fiber; and drug varietals, which are used for their psychotropic effects or medicinal benefits.

Hemp Varietals

Cannabis sativa spp. *sativa*: Narrow-leaf hemp (NLH), nonpsychoactive, used for food, fuel, fiber, and, more recently, for CBD products

Early Range: Europe

Growth Characteristics and Description: A loosely branched plant with thin leaves, sometimes very narrow and spindly (with very few branches). This species is often grown very close together when it will be used for fiber. Preventing the plant from branching out horizontally focuses its energy on vertical growth, producing tall plants with long fibers. Its flowers are generally loose and not dense.

Cannabis indica ssp. *chinensis*: Broad-leaf hemp (BLH), nonpsychoactive, broad leaves, used for food, fuel, fiber, and, more recently, CBD products

Early Range: China, Korea, Japan, and Southeast Asia

Growth Characteristics and Description: A densely branching plant with wide leaves and a shorter growing season. Its flowers are dense; its plants are shorter than those of other varieties.

Drug Varietals

Cannabis indica spp. *afghanica*: Broad-leaf drug (BLD), what people currently call *Cannabis indica*

Early Range: Northern Afghanistan and Pakistan

Growth Characteristics and Description: A densely branching plant with wide leaves and a short growing season. It is found in colder climates. Its flowers are dense; its plants are shorter than those of other varieties.

Cannabis indica spp. *indica*: Narrow-leaf drug (NLD), what people currently call *Cannabis sativa*

Early Range: South and Southeast Asia, and Middle East

Growth Characteristics and Description: A loosely branched plant with thin leaves and a long growing season. It likes warmer climates with a longer growing season. Its flowers have a loose structure.

Cannabis ruderalis spp. *ruderalis*: These plants are what people know as autoflowers (see page 6).

Early Range: Northern Central Asia

Growth Characteristics and Description: A short and often unbranched plant with thin, small leaves that have three to five leaflets. It flowers according to age and is not photoperiod-dependent. It has low amounts of THC and CBD and is often used to breed autoflowering cultivars.

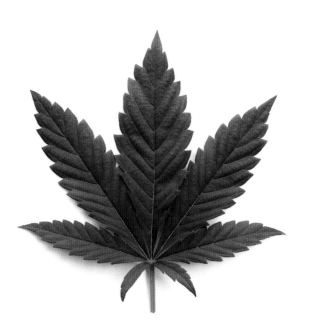

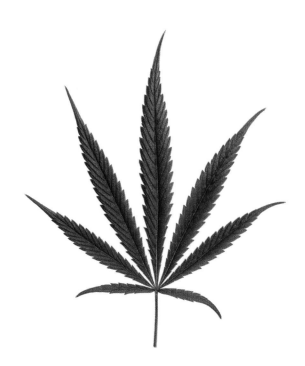

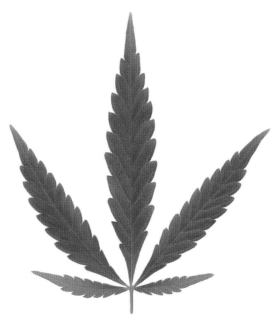

These leaves come from the following varieties of cannabis, *starting from the top left moving clockwise:* broad-leaf drug plant (*Cannabis indica* spp. *afghanica*), narrow-leaf drug plant (*Cannabis indica* spp. *indica*), and ruderalis plant (*Cannabis ruderalis* spp. *ruderalis*).

CANNABIS VARIETIES

In this section, you will find information that will help you when researching the varieties of cannabis that will best suit your needs. It may be hard for the new or inexperienced grower to know where to start when looking at the multitude of options available. This will help you understand how cannabis is classified and for what reason.

Cultivars

When speaking about cannabis, people often refer to *strains* when differentiating between different varieties of the plant. A more accurate word to use would be *cultivar*, which is short for "cultivated variety." A cultivar is a plant that humans have selected and intentionally bred for certain desirable characteristics and maintained through cultivation. When a cultivar breeds true and its genetics are stable, these characteristics will appear in the next generation. You can also maintain a cultivar by taking cuttings, a process called cloning (see page 122). Cloning is practiced extensively in the cannabis industry.

Breeders will select parent plants for a wide variety of reasons. These reasons may range from a plant's flavor and terpene profile, cannabinoid content, plant structure, early finishing, and disease resistance—the list goes on and on. There are an infinite number of possibilities when it comes to breeding new cultivars, and new ones are being created all the time. Northern Lights, Blueberry, Manitoba Poison, 88 G-13 Hashplant, Sour Diesel, and Gelato—these are just a few examples of cannabis cultivars you can find.

Chemovars

The term *chemovar* is used to describe the presence of chemical constituents in a specific cultivar as well as their quantity and potency. These constituents include terpenes, flavonoids, cannabinoids, and more. By measuring the chemical constituents in a plant, we can differentiate between the chemistries of different cultivars

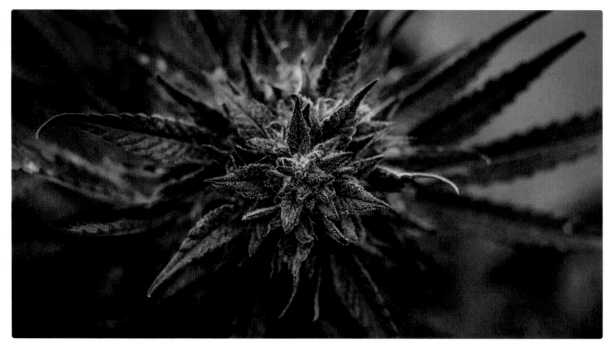

The Thorsberry is a hybrid cannabis cultivar known for its striking reddish purple leaves. It has been used for pain management, post-traumatic stress disorder, depression, insomnia, stress, and nausea.

and know the physiological effects each one will trigger. When it comes to using cannabis as medicine, having this knowledge allows for more precise dosing, which, in turn, can provide reproducible results.

Whereas anyone can change the name of a cultivar, the chemical makeup of specific chemovars is usually static. By measuring the level of active cannabinoids, such as THC and CBD, and terpenes, we can gain a better understanding of how to predict the physiological effects that a cultivar will have. This is helpful for patients who want to treat specific ailments or conditions by making it easier to ensure that they are receiving the same medicinal compounds each time they use cannabis and the best ones for their condition. For example, it has been found that one way to potentially improve the efficacy of THC (as well as lower the adverse reactions to it) is to choose cannabis chemovars that contain some CBD and have a terpenoid-rich profile to produce the best results.

Many cannabis cultivars can be broadly classified into three chemovar categories:

Type I: THC-dominant. Most of the current cannabis available in the medical and recreational marketplaces of North America and Europe falls into this category. These plants have large percentages of THC and very low percentages of CBD.

Type II: Contains a balanced ratio of THC and CBD. These chemovars will have close to equal parts of CBD and THC. Studies have shown that cannabis with a 1:1 ratio of THC to CBD consistently shows the best results when used as medicine for a number of ailments.

Type III: CBD-dominant. In the past decade, as more research has come out about the therapeutic benefits of CBD, there has been an increased interest and demand for more cultivars that have a higher CBD content. This has led breeders to select for this trait and increase the availability of CBD-dominant cannabis.

Many cultivars, especially those available on the legal market, are now being tested in laboratories to determine their chemical constituents. This information is being compiled and made available to the public. Many labs will also test a sample of your own homegrown cannabis for a fee. With testing, you can be sure of what you'll find in each plant and gain a clearer understanding of how you will react when you use it, though this may not be an economical option for every home grower.

You can always use your personal experiences with smoking, vaping, or ingesting your cannabis or a product made with your cannabis to guide you instead. It will take time, but with practice and careful observation you will gain the necessary skills to confidently predict how each cultivar of cannabis affects you.

I recommend keeping a journal and recording your experiences each time you use cannabis. It will serve as an invaluable tool for gaining a more in-depth look at how cannabis works for you. Start by describing the smell, taste, and how it makes you feel when you consume it. You can look online using the keywords "cannabis journal template" and find a number of sample pages with a series of questions to guide your observations.

Landrace Varieties

Landrace varieties of cannabis have evolved in a specific geographic location in relative isolation over a long period and have been tended to by local growers and farmers. These cultivars have adapted to local environmental conditions and are often considered to have a more balanced level of compounds and a more predictable effect when taken internally. Because they have grown in the same bioregion for hundreds and

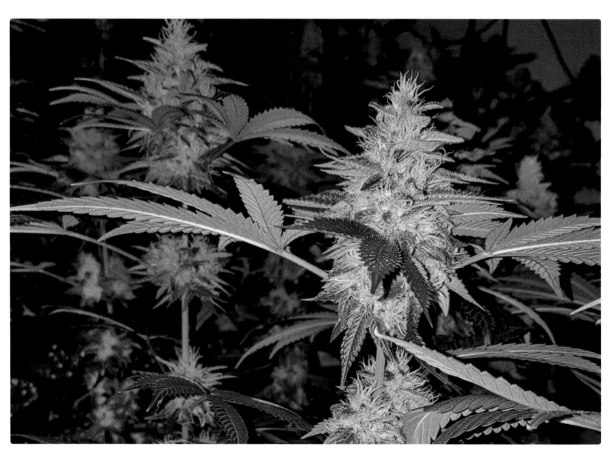

This Afghani is a landrace that has adapted to the climate found in the mountains of Afghanistan. It was used to breed many modern cultivars now being grown in North America and beyond.

sometimes thousands of years, they tend to be more likely to breed true.

There are very few true landraces left in the world, as almost all species of cannabis have been hybridized, especially in the West. It was only in the late 1960s and early 1970s that many "exotic" landrace strains made their way to North America. These landraces formed the building blocks of our modern cannabis cultivars, and many were often named after the regions that they came from.

EXAMPLES OF LANDRACES

Afghanistan: Pure Afghan, Hindu Kush, Afghani, Mazar-I-Sharif

Brazil: Santa Maria

Central Africa: Congolese

China: Kumaoni

Colombia: Colombian Gold

Egypt: Sinai

India: Kerala, Mysuru, Chennai

Jamaica: Lamb's Bread

Japan: Hokkaido

Lebanon: Lebanese

Mexico: Acapulco Gold, Oaxacan

Morocco: Ketama

Nepal: Kumaoni, Nepalese

Pakistan: Pakistani, Pakistani Chitral Kush, Tirah

Panama: Panama Red

South Africa: Durban Poison

Swaziland: Swazi Gold

Syria: Syrian

Thailand: Highland Thai

Benefits of Cannabis

The following chart lists the effects that cannabis can provide and the cannabinoids, terpenes, and cultivars that will produce those effects. These are just some of the many ways that cannabis is being used medicinally right now. As more research comes out, we may discover more applications. This is by no means an exhaustive list and is meant merely as a starting point. Many cultivars can be used for these conditions, and some will work better than others, as each person is unique and will modulate the effects of the cannabis differently.

USES FOR CANNABIS

Use	Cannabinoids	Terpenes	Cultivars
Analgesic (reduces pain)	THC, CBD, cannabigerol (CBG), tetrahydrocannabivarin (THCV), cannabichromene (CBC), cannabinol (CBN), cannabidiolic acid (CBDA)	Caryophyllene, humulene, linalool, myrcene, pinene	Most high-THC and high-CBD varieties, including Skunk, OG Kush, Cookies, Kryptonite, Harlequin, Rainbow Gumeez, ACDC, and Blackberry Kush
Anticonvulsant	CBD, THC, CBDV, CBDA	Linalool, terpinolene	Charlotte's Web, Lavender, Harlequin, Critical Mass, Headband, Amnesia Haze
Antioxidant	THC, THCA, CBD, CBDA	Caryophyllene, pinene, terpinolene	Most cultivars are considered to have antioxidant properties. Look for ones with the cannabinoids and terpenes listed in this row.
Anti-cancer	High THC, CBD, CBG, CBC, THCA, CBDA	Humulene, myrcene, limonene, pinene, terpinolene	Tangerine Dream, Gelato, Blue Dream
Antidepressant	THC, CBD	Caryophyllene, limonene, linalool	Gelato, Tangie, Blue Dream, Super Silver Haze, Chernobyl
Antiemetic (manages nausea/vomiting)	THC, CBD, CBDA	Caryophyllene, limonene	Super Lemon Haze, Blueberry Diesel, Northern Lights, Sour Strawberry, Durban Poison
Anti-insomnia	High THC, THCA, CBN, CBG	Terpinolene, linalool, myrcene (at levels above 0.5%)	Hindu Kush, Bubba Kush, Grape Ape, Purps, Lavender Kush

Use	Cannabinoids	Terpenes	Cultivars
Anti-spasmodic	THC, CBD, THCV, THCA	Limonene, linalool, myrcene	AK-47, Grape Ape, Sensi Star, Lavender, CBD Critical Mass, Face Off OG
Anxiolytic (anti-anxiety)	CBD, THC, CBC, THCV	Caryophyllene, limonene, myrcene, pinene, terpinolene	Purple Orange CBD, ACDC, Cherry Pie, Cannatonic, Harlequin, Remedy, White Widow
Appetite stimulant	THC, CBG	Caryophyllene, myrcene	Most high-THC cultivars will provoke this response, including OG Kush, Lemon Kush, Cheese, and Cookies.
Creative stimulant	THC, THCV	Limonene, pinene	Sour Diesel, Old Afghani, Jack Herer, Tangerine Dream, Candyland, Skunk
End-of-life comfort (both physical and spiritual comfort)	CBD for distress (daytime use), THC for pain and better sleep	N/A	The best cultivar will vary depending on the individual.
Focusing agent	THC, THCV	Limonene, pinene	Jack Herer, NYC Diesel
Neurogenesis	THC, CBC, CBD, THCA	Caryophyllene, limonene, linalool, pinene	Any cultivars with the terpenes and cannabinoids listed.
Neuroprotective	CBD, THC, THCA, CBDA	Caryophyllene, pinene	Jack Herer, AK-47, White Widow, Girl Scout Cookies

LIFE CYCLE OF CANNABIS

Once a cannabis seed is planted, it will sprout within a few days under the right conditions and the new plant will break the soil and begin to grow toward the sun within 1–2 weeks (older seeds may take a little longer). It then enters its first stage of life—the seedling stage. At this point, the young plant is beginning to grow leaves and direct its upward growth toward the source of light. This stage will last for approximately 2–3 weeks, at which time your plant will become larger and show four to six sets of branches.

Your plant will then enter the vegetative stage and will begin to grow vigorously. It can quite easily grow 2 inches (5 cm) or more per day. When growing indoors, your plants can stay in this vegetative growth stage for years as long as they are receiving 18 hours of light per day. Outdoors, in a northern latitude, your plants will spend anywhere from 2 to 5 months in the vegetative stage, depending on where you live, the amount of daylight you receive, and the specific cultivar that you are growing. Some plants will naturally stay in the vegetative stage for longer than others. Autoflowering cannabis may spend

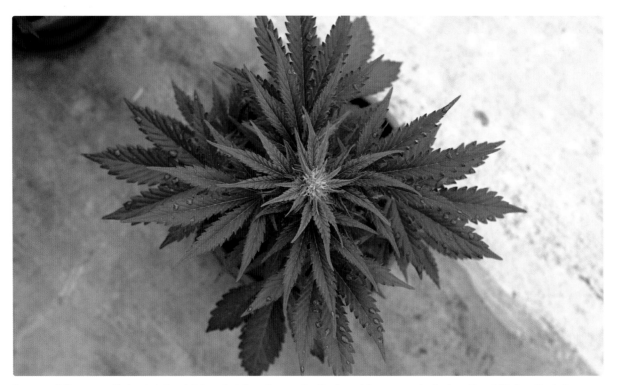

Because autoflower cannabis is not photoperiod-dependent, it can be a great option for aspiring growers who live in northern latitudes with shorter growing seasons, have limited space, or are looking for a beginner-friendly plant to grow.

as little as 2–3 weeks in a vegetative state before they begin to flower. If you plan to take cuttings to produce clones from your plants, you will want to do this while the plant is still in a vegetative state.

When grown outdoors, your plants will enter the flowering stage once the days begin to shorten. This can happen anywhere from the third week of July to the first or second week of August in much of North America. Most cultivars will flower for a minimum of 4–6 weeks before they are mature, with some longer flowering varieties taking as long as 3–4 months. On average, most cannabis cultivars will take 6–8 weeks to flower and reach maturity when grown outdoors.

Cannabis is wind-pollinated. This is one reason the male plants often grow more quickly and taller, and start to flower a little earlier than female plants. This allows the wind to carry pollen to the pistils of the female flowers more easily. Each pistil or "hair" can receive pollen and produce a single seed, and a well-pollinated female plant can potentially produce thousands and thousands of seeds!

If pollinated, seeds will take approximately 4–6 weeks to mature under ideal conditions. Cannabis is an annual plant, meaning that it will naturally grow to maturity and die within one growing cycle. Once it has flowered, it will die back and not come back to life the following year. Overall, many of you can expect that your plants will grow from April or May until October or November before their growing season comes to a close.

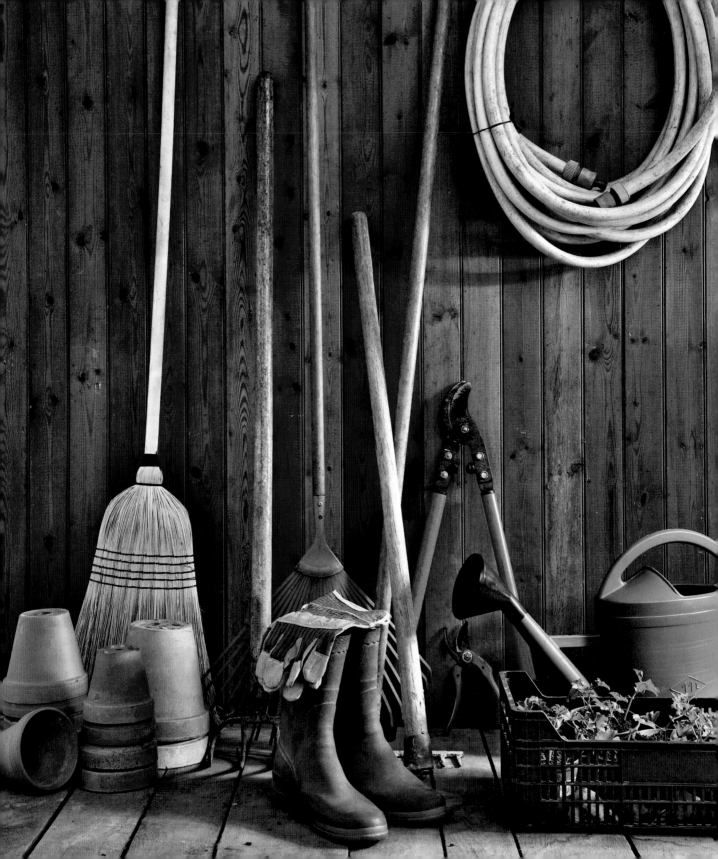

CHAPTER 2

< Tools & Equipment >

There is a proper tool for every job, and this conventional wisdom very much applies to growing cannabis. Although the only things that your plants need are sun, soil, and water, there are some tools and equipment that will make the planning, germination, growing, harvesting, and storing processes much easier. Some of these items will be vital to growing your cannabis plants, while others will make your gardening life more efficient and help your plants to grow more quickly, and become stronger and healthier.

FINDING YOUR TOOLS & EQUIPMENT

This chapter describes many tools and equipment that are commonly used to grow cannabis, but you may not need all the things that are listed. It is best to use this information as a reference rather than a "must-have" list. You may find that you already have many of the items described or something around your house that will work similarly. That's great—use what you have. It also does not hurt to source used items before buying new ones. Choosing used items will save you money and is better for the planet. You may be surprised by the quality of the secondhand tools that are sold at heavily discounted prices.

If you are going to buy new, beware of cheap items because they are often cheap for a reason. Many inexpensive tools are poorly made and will not last. I have a nice pair of secateurs that cost close to $100, but they are more than twenty years old. Sure, they were expensive, but the high upfront cost became a very small investment after twenty years' worth of use. Do your research on every product you buy, and ask yourself whether you really need it and what benefits this new tool or piece of equipment will give you. What are the warranties, and how long will they last? Is it more efficient to use this item, and will it save you time and money now or in the future?

LEFT Having a place to store your tools and equipment is just as important as investing in high-quality items. It is important to clean your tools after use and designate a spot for each item.

< 19 >

Whenever possible, support small and local businesses. By buying from your local businesses, your money supports not only the small business owners but also their employees. The income that they earn will also be spent and invested in other shops and companies in your area. Although it is easy to purchase everything you need online, many businesses would not last without our support, and our local economies would suffer.

Many of the tools listed in this chapter should be available from your local garden center or nursery, but if you have a local hydroponic or grow store, I recommend visiting it. Most large urban centers will have one in their area. Even if you live in a state where growing cannabis is not legal, there is most likely one of these stores around selling specialized equipment that you can use. Even if you do not purchase anything from these stores, you may find it helpful to look at various tools and equipment, such as lights, in person, and talk to a knowledgeable staff member who can answer your questions and give you advice on particular products. If you choose to patronize a specialty store, beware of the markup that is often added to cannabis-specific tools and equipment. With a little research, you may find some of the same tools at a hardware store for a lot less. The cannabis industry is notorious for charging premium prices for products that you can find elsewhere much less expensively.

There is one last piece of advice that I want to give: It is a good idea to start small for your first grow and scale up from there. If you try to do too much without the proper experience, you may be setting yourself up for failure and picking up tools that you don't need. Try growing a few plants from seed to harvest and get the feel for it before expanding your garden,

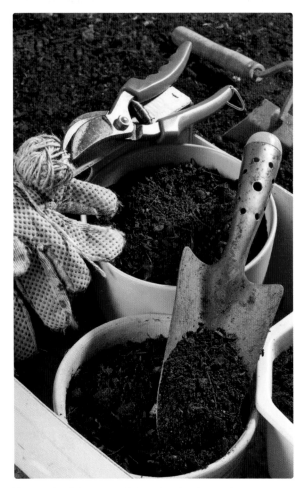

You may already have many of the tools and equipment that you'll need. Growing cannabis requires many of the same items needed for vegetable or flower gardening, and using what you have will be easier on your budget.

selecting just the tools and equipment that are crucial for your first grow. For your subsequent grows, you can pick up any additional items that will make your gardening experience more efficient and effective. Once you gain some experience and get to know the cannabis plant, it will be easier for you to determine which items are essential for you and your personal growing conditions and which items may not be crucial or needed at all.

THE ESSENTIALS

The tools and equipment listed below are arranged in the approximate order that you need them throughout the season. Many of the items are useful, no matter where you are growing your cannabis, but there are some items that are needed only if you are growing exclusively indoors or outdoors (see "The Essentials at a Glance," below). Remember, you do not need everything on this list.

THE ESSENTIALS AT A GLANCE

For outdoor and indoor growing:

- Cell packs and propagation trays
- Pots
- Potting soil
- Water buckets
- Min/max thermometer hygrometer
- Spray bottle
- Plant supports
- Measuring cups
- Air pump or aerator
- Strainer
- Funnel
- Pruning shears (handheld secateurs)
- Trimming scissors
- Rubbing alcohol
- Razor blade
- Gardening gloves
- Long-sleeved shirt
- Rubber gloves
- String
- Drying screens and racks
- Kitchen scale
- Glass jars or resealable plastic bags
- Jewelry loupe, hand lens, or magnifying glass

For outdoor growing only:

- Shovel or trowel

For indoor growing only:

- Humidity dome
- Heating mat
- Grow lights
- pH meter and/or litmus paper
- Trowel

Depending on the setup of your indoor grow space, you may need additional equipment, such as fans or dehumidifiers. To determine whether this is the case, review the information on maintaining indoor growing conditions on pages 49–63.

Cell Packs & Propagation Trays

Cell packs are small plastic inserts used to germinate seedlings or hold clones. Each pack generally contains four, six, or nine individual cells. The cell packs are held in a propagation tray. Propagation trays make it easy to store and move your seedlings. Some propagation trays will catch any extra water runoff that drips out of the cells. You can also use them to hold pots. The number of cell packs and trays you need will be determined by how many plants you want to grow. In most cases, you will just need one or two trays and the corresponding number of cell packs to fill them. You can reuse both the trays and cell packs each year.

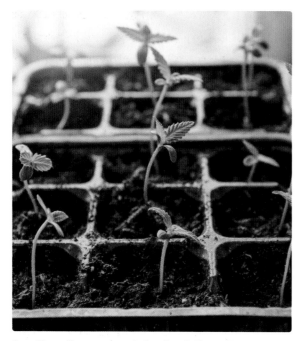

Cannabis seedlings grow in a plastic cell pack. These cell packs also make it convenient to transport and transplant many young plants at once, and take up a small amount of space.

Pots

For plants grown in the ground outdoors, I suggest buying a 4-inch (10 cm) and 1-gallon (3.8 L) pot with drainage holes for each of your plants. This way, you can transplant seedlings and clones from your cell pack twice: once into a 4-inch pot and once into a 1-gallon pot. If you plan to grow your plants indoors or keep them in pots outside, you will want to have some pots in larger sizes, such as 5-, 10-, or 20-gallon (19, 38, or 76 L) containers, to accommodate full-size plants. You may want to explore fabric pots for plants that you are going to grow outdoors in containers. They may prevent your plants from becoming root-bound, are lightweight, and dry out more quickly, helping you avoid the effects of overwatering.

Potting Soil

When planting seeds and clones, you will want to have some seed-starting soil on hand. You want your seed-starting mix to be light and full of organic matter. It should stay moist and lofty, and avoid becoming hard and dense when it dries out. As you transplant your plants into larger pots, you will also need a soil mix that has all the nutrients your plants will need as they grow bigger. (For more information about soil mixes, including recipes for homemade mixes, see page 81.)

Buckets

It will be good to have one or two 5-gallon (19-L) buckets that can be used for watering your plants as well as brewing plant and compost teas. You can also use them to mix soil and complete many other tasks. If you have a lot of plants, you may want to consider getting larger buckets so that you can store and deliver a larger amount of water more easily.

Min/Max Thermometer Hygrometer

For the indoor grower, a thermometer that records the minimum and maximum temperatures of your garden and measures humidity will be invaluable. It will allow you to constantly

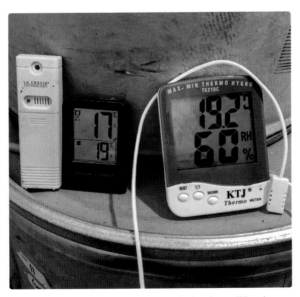

A min/max thermometer hygrometer for monitoring the conditions in your growing environment is crucial for indoor and greenhouse growers. The black device shown here comes with a remote sensor (*the white device on the left*) that can be moved closer to the area that you want to monitor.

monitor your conditions, detect fluctuations in temperature and humidity, and show you how the temperature and humidity are changing in your grow space when you are not there. The minimum and maximum readings will be key to discovering when something is off. Many stores carry these devices, and they are a small investment to make for the peace of mind that they will bring.

Spray Bottle

A spray bottle will be important to have around for both indoor and outdoor growers. You can use it to foliar-feed your plants with nutrients such as plant teas (see page 132). It will also come in handy for applying natural insecticides, should you have an outbreak of pests, such as thrips, mites, or aphids. You can find inexpensive 1-quart (1-L) spray bottles at your local garden center or the gardening sections of other stores. If you increase the size of your garden, you can look into larger, more advanced sprayers. These will cost more, but they will allow you to cover a larger area in less time. It is important to clean your sprayer and bottle thoroughly at the end of each use and before filling it with another liquid. Having a couple of spray bottles on hand for different liquids is a good idea.

Plant Supports

Supporting your cannabis plants is very important (see page 147) and will give them a better opportunity to reach their full potential. When your plants are young and small, a simple piece of bamboo, a wooden stake, or a tomato cage will suffice. As they get bigger and develop more branches, you will want to consider using wire fences, cages, or trellis netting for extra support. Though some plants may have the structural integrity to hold themselves upright on their own, I recommend that all new growers support all of their plants until they gain the experience to determine which plants need it and which ones don't. The last thing you want to see is your immature flower branches toppled over and broken prematurely from a strong wind or rainstorm.

Measuring Cups

Measuring cups will allow you to add precise amounts of fertilizers or soil amendments to your water or soil. They will also be helpful when you make the recipes for homemade fertilizer and soil mixing. I recommend having cups in a few different sizes, including one that measures liquids in small milliliter increments between 1 and 50 milliliters as well as a one-cup measuring device. They do not have to be fancy, as long as they can accurately measure the ingredients.

Air Pump or Aerator

Air pumps or aerators are used to oxygenate your compost, manure, and plant teas. By forcing air into the water in these mixtures, they prevent harmful anaerobic bacteria from growing,

maintain the proper environment for good bacteria, and infuse the liquid with oxygen. Pet and fish stores often carry these pumps for use in fish tanks, and you can also find them at your local grow store or online. You will want an air pump that can handle the amount of tea you plan to brew. For a setup with a 5-gallon (19-L) bucket, you can get away with a smaller pump, while a setup with a 50-gallon (189-L) barrel will need a larger one.

Strainer

A large wire-mesh strainer will separate plant material from your plant teas (unless you used a burlap bag to act as a tea bag). Removing this material from plant teas makes it easier to water your plants with a tea solution and will slow down the decomposition process that may lead to the formation of anaerobic bacteria. You do not need a specific kind of strainer as long as it can filter out the plant material. If you are using 5-gallon (19-L) buckets, it is ideal to find one that securely fits over its top.

Funnel

A funnel will help you transfer liquids from one bucket to another and can be used with a strainer. You can also use it to fill up spray bottles. The best size and shape for you will be determined by the quantity of liquid you are transferring as well as the size of the buckets or containers you are using. Funnels can be found in the kitchen section of many stores, at kitchen supply stores, and online.

Pruning Shears (Handheld Secateurs)

A good pair of pruning shears allow you to chop your plants down with ease and efficiency during harvesting. As their name suggests, they can also be used for pruning. Cannabis and hemp are known for their incredibly strong, fibrous stalks, which can be hard to cut through. You can always use a knife or a saw to cut down your plants, but neither of those tools is anywhere near as efficient as a sharp pair of handheld secateurs.

Trimming Scissors

A high-quality pair of handheld scissors is essential for trimming your flowers after harvest. Be sure to choose a pair that is comfortable to hold. You can find them at your local grower supply store or online.

Rubbing Alcohol

You will use rubbing alcohol to disinfect and clean tools. It will prevent you from spreading mold or disease if one of your plants is sick. When you are trimming, the rubbing alcohol will aid in cleaning the resin that will inevitably build up on the blades of your scissors and keep them from

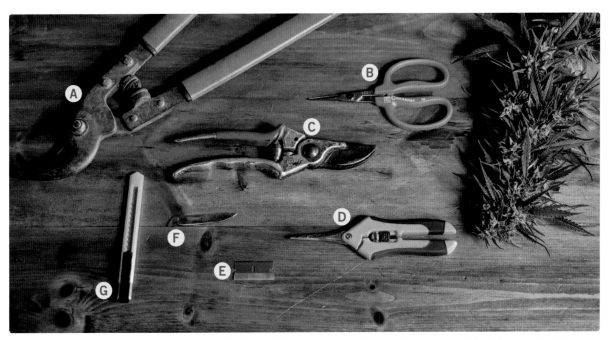

Growing cannabis will require tools that can cut tough stalks, delicate sugar leaves, and everything in between. Pictured here, *starting from the top left and moving clockwise*, are long-handled pruning shears (*A*), trimming scissors (*B*), handheld pruners (*C*), spring-loaded trimming shears (*D*), a razor blade (*E*), blade for a craft knife (*F*), and a utility knife (*G*). I have been using the handheld pruners for twenty years.

working effectively. Some growers have several pairs of trimming scissors to maintain speed and efficiency while manicuring their flowers. They will have one pair soaking in alcohol while they use the other pair and then rotate.

Razor Blade

A sharp blade, such as a razor, is very important when taking cuttings for cloning. You want to get a nice, clean, even cut, and having a sharp blade will make this process more efficient as well as increase the number of cuttings that successfully form roots and turn into young plants.

Gardening Gloves

Gardening gloves are helpful for people who do not want to get their hands dirty when working with soil and can protect your hands when you're working with sharp tools or from rocks in your garden. They will also keep dirt from entering any cuts or scrapes you may have on your hands and limit the potential of possible infection.

Long-Sleeved Shirt

When harvesting, I recommend wearing a long-sleeved shirt, unless you want to be covered with sticky resin from your flowers. Some people will experience contact dermatitis from the resin that cannabis produces. An easy way to avoid this experience is to cover up. You do not need a specific kind of shirt, just something that prevents your skin from coming in contact with the resin.

Rubber Gloves

If you experience contact dermatitis from cannabis or you want to keep your hands resin-free, it is a good idea to have some tight-fitting rubber gloves to use when you are harvesting and trimming your flowers. The tighter they are, the better. Tighter gloves make it easier for you to feel and manipulate the flowers, especially when trimming. Disposable latex gloves work well for this, but they do end up in a landfill so they are not the most environmentally friendly. I find that you can often reuse them a few times if you are careful when taking them off.

String

You will use string made from a strong material, such as nylon or mason's twine, to create lines to hang cannabis for drying. You want string that is strong enough to support your branches and will not stretch when weighed down by plants. If the string stretches, your plants will slide to the middle and will not be evenly spaced, preventing adequate air from flowing between the branches. Some growers use trellis netting (see page 148) to hang their plants, instead of string.

Drying Screens and Racks

After harvest, I usually hang my plants to dry on strings or lines (see photo on page 178), but there are inevitably some smaller buds that will need to be put on some kind of drying rack or screen.

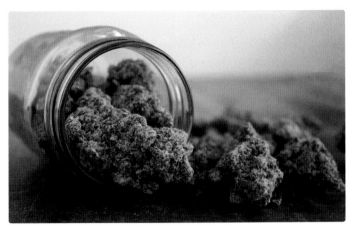
Glass jars can be an ideal option for storing dried and cured buds as they do not react to the chemical compounds in cannabis, or absorb or release odors.

You can make your own drying racks by building a wooden frame and securing some fiberglass mesh to it or using old window screens, which can often be found for free or quite inexpensively. You can also try using expandable drying baskets that can be hung from the ceiling. These often have multiple tiers on which you can spread out your buds. Whatever you choose to use, make sure your screen or rack allows air to flow on all sides of the buds so that they dry evenly and do not grow mold.

Kitchen Scale

A kitchen scale will allow you to weigh your harvest once it is dried to see how much dried flower comes from each of your plants. It is not an essential tool, but it will enable you to see which plants produced the most. You will also use a kitchen scale to weigh cannabis should you decide to make medicinal or wellness products from it.

Glass Jars or Resealable Plastic Bags

You will need to have some bags or containers for storing your harvest once it has dried. Glass jars are always my first choice. They come in many different sizes and can be reused for years. However, jars may not be practical with a large harvest. If this is the case for you, then you will want to consider using food-safe plastic bags to store your flowers. Poultry bags work well. You can also use many of the resealable plastic bags available at your local grocery store. Try storing some of your flowers in glass and some in plastic (if you do not have enough glass jars) and see if you can notice a difference in quality after long-term storage.

Shovel or Trowel

For outdoor growers, a shovel is an essential tool for digging holes, mixing soil in a bucket or wheelbarrow, as well as applying compost, manure, and soil amendments to your garden beds. A trowel can also be helpful for the outdoor grower, but it is nowhere near as important as a shovel. Trowels are better suited for indoor growers and can be used to transplant plants and add amendments to pots.

Humidity Dome

Humidity domes are helpful for both cloning and germinating seeds. They are placed over your propagation trays to help trap humidity and keep the soil in your cell packs from drying out. They can be purchased fairly inexpensively from your local grow store or garden center. If you would like to use a humidity dome for cloning, be sure to get the tall domes that are around 6–8 inches (15–20 cm) tall.

Heating Mat

Heating mats are used to germinate seeds or root clones. They are not essential, but they can help improve your germination rate. You place them beneath your propagation trays or pots to warm them a few degrees above the ambient air temperature. (Some mats will also keep the surface a few degrees cooler than the surrounding air temperature.) The extra warmth can help speed up the germination or rooting process, especially in a cooler environment. Some heating mats will come with a built-in thermostat.

Grow Lights

If you will cultivate your plants indoors, consider purchasing different types of grow lights. Fluorescent or LED lights work best for young plants. For plants in vegetative growth or the flowering stage, you may want to purchase a metal halide, high-pressure sodium, or high-quality LED light. For more information on lighting for indoor growing, see page 50.

pH Meter and Litmus Paper

Though pH meters and litmus paper are not really necessary if you're using living soils (page 67), they are handy tools. Having the ability to check the pH of your water or the water that runs out of the bottom of your pot is important for indoor growers who raise their plants in pots. The readings can be especially helpful for diagnosing potential problems with your plants or growing environment. Some pH meters will also measure water temperature, electrical conductivity (EC), and total dissolved solids (TDS).

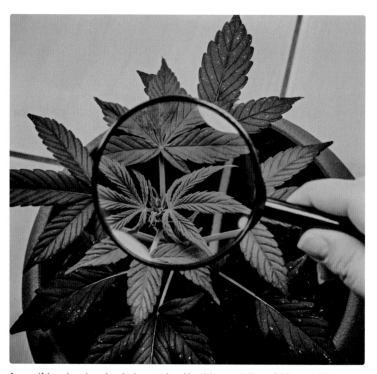

A magnifying glass (or a jewelry loupe or hand lens) is especially useful for examining trichomes, which will help you determine whether your buds are mature enough to harvest. It is also handy for detecting pests on the leaves and stems of your plants.

Jewelry Loupe, Hand Lens, or Magnifying Glass

You will use these items to look at the trichomes on your flowers when you are deciding whether they are ready to harvest. This will allow you to time your harvest optimally and collect mature buds at their peak potency. These tools also come in handy for inspecting your plants for pests and diseases, and identifying insects.

MAINTAINING YOUR TOOLS & EQUIPMENT

Once you acquire some tools and equipment for growing your plants, I recommend dedicating a space to store them and not using this space for anything else. When you have finished using an item, return it to that location. This will allow you to easily locate and pick out the proper tools for each job and keep them arranged in an organized fashion. This space may be a shelf, a cupboard, or even a plastic tote with a lid.

Always clean and sterilize tools with alcohol after using them (especially cutting tools that may have come in contact with a diseased plant). Make sure your tools are dry before storing them away in order to avoid rust and harmful pathogens or bacteria from forming on them. If you take care of your tools and equipment, you can be sure that they will be there for you when you need them.

FAQS & TROUBLESHOOTING

Q: Why are cannabis-specific products, tools, and equipment so expensive? What do I do if I'm on a budget?

A: Part of the answer to this question revolves around the fact that cannabis retailers and equipment companies operate within a niche market. Therefore, they try to get a premium price for their products. I think the other reason for the high prices has to do with the fact that during the prohibition years, most people who grew cannabis needed to shop almost exclusively at grow shops. There were not many other options, and you had to pay the high price for products and equipment that you needed.

If you're on a budget, I suggest that you always shop around and look for the same or similar tools and equipment at nonspecialty stores. Garden centers, nurseries, and animal feed stores could all be good places to get a better deal. Before you go shopping, always check what you or your friends may have on hand. A lot of people have extra gardening tools that they no longer use and may be willing to part with. There is nothing wrong with secondhand or upcycled items. In fact, the use of secondhand tools complements the principles of regenerative farming, and I encourage you to do so.

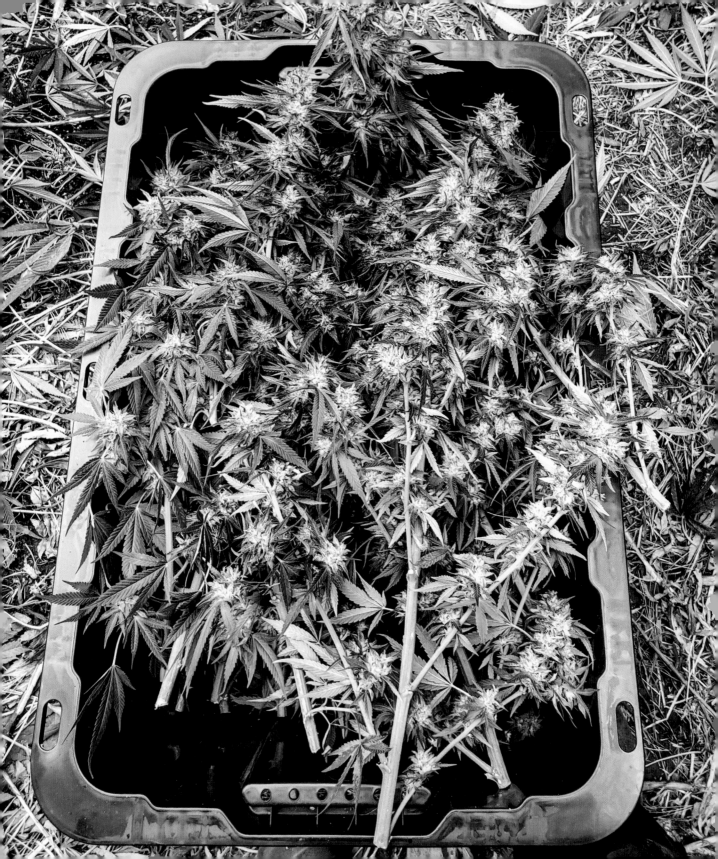

CHAPTER 3

< Planning Your Garden >

Each grower has many choices to make when cultivating cannabis. You will want to consider whether you will grow your cannabis plants indoors or outdoors. You will need to determine whether you have enough space or the proper location to grow your plants. Putting a little time and thought into these decisions is important. In this chapter, we will look into some of the factors to take into account when planning your garden and discuss the pros and cons of growing your plants indoors or outdoors.

EVALUATING YOUR GROWING ENVIRONMENT

Cannabis is a very versatile plant and has adapted to many different growing conditions around the world. It can thrive in the harsh, high mountain conditions of Afghanistan and Pakistan as well as the humid tropical rain forests of South America and Southeast Asia. This is a good thing for cannabis growers. It means that with a little searching, you should be able to find a cultivar that will grow well outdoors in your area. Even if you live in the Far North, there are now autoflower varieties that can be grown from seed to harvest in sixty days or less. If you want to grow indoors, you have even more possibilities. You can grow cannabis indoors in any region in the world as long as you have access to a power source and some lights.

It is up to individual growers to choose how and where they will grow cannabis based on their available resources, preferences, and environmental conditions. Let's take a look at some questions that you should ask yourself when making these decisions.

LEFT Careful planning and an honest evaluation of the growing conditions, resources, and space available to you are an important first step to ensuring a bountiful harvest.

< 31 >

Is it legal to grow cannabis for personal or medical use in your area? How many plants can you legally grow?

It is important to make sure that you check your provincial, state, and federal laws before growing cannabis. In Canada, cannabis was federally legalized for recreational use in 2018. As of this writing, you are legally allowed to grow four plants per household in all Canadian provinces (with the exception of Quebec and Manitoba). To grow more than four plants, you need to acquire a medical cannabis prescription from a doctor or a nurse practitioner for an approved condition and then apply for a permit through Health Canada.

In the United States, things are a little different. Cannabis is currently still illegal on a federal level, but it has been legalized for medical use in thirty-four states as well as for recreational use in fifteen states and the District of Columbia. In order to acquire a state-sanctioned medical permit, you will need to have an ailment that has been diagnosed by a physician that is also on your state's list of qualified conditions. This permit will allow you to purchase and use cannabis, and some states will allow you to grow your own medical cannabis with this permit. In the states that have legalized recreational cannabis, you may be allowed to grow a certain number of cannabis plants for personal use. Because each state has different laws and regulations, it is very important for you to do your research and make

sure that you are abiding by all the rules set out by your state government.

How much time do you have, and how much money do you wish to spend?

To achieve the best results, as well as the best quality of cannabis possible, make sure that you set aside enough time and money. Taking care of cannabis will require a similar amount of time as planting and growing a small vegetable garden. That may be as little as one or two hours a week for 2–4 plants or many hours a week for a larger garden.

Growing cannabis indoors will take a similar amount of time as growing plants outdoors, but you will need to devote extra time for watering and monitoring your lights and environmental conditions. Indoor growing is also generally more expensive than growing outdoors, as there are costs involved in using electricity and purchasing lights, timers, exhaust and intake fans, nutrients, and fertilizers. You might also need to purchase a grow tent or build a space in which to grow your plants. Setting up a grow space in your house or apartment will typically cost you approximately $500–$1,000, sometimes more, depending on what equipment you need to purchase.

No matter what growing method you choose, you can keep your costs low by using tools, equipment, and inputs (such as amendments and fertilizers) that you already have at your disposal, as well as following the tips and advice given in this book.

Do you have access to a place to grow some plants outdoors?

You can grow cannabis in your backyard, on a farm, on a balcony, on a deck, and more. Perhaps you have a family member or a friend who would let you grow your plants on their property. Even though cannabis plants can grow quite large, you may be surprised how you can prune and train them to fit into a smaller space.

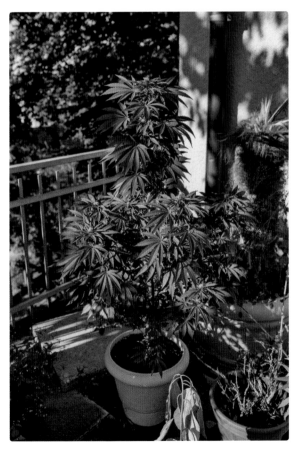

Even a container placed on an outdoor balcony can work as a growing space as long as your cannabis has sufficient room to grow and has access to water and sunlight.

If you grow cannabis outside, will it have access to soil, water, and sunshine?

If you have a backyard or access to a plot of land, you can grow your plants directly in your native soil without adding any amendments, fertilizers, or other inputs. I do, however, recommend that you add at least some of the inputs or make some of the recipes in this book.

Water is generally easy to come by, either directly from your tap or from a well, pond, or other local water source. If you live in a dry area (or want to conserve groundwater), you may want to look into setting up a rainwater catchment system where you can collect and store rainwater. This can be done simply by attaching a rain barrel to your eaves trough or by setting up a more complex system of pipes and filters.

Luckily, sunshine is free and is the ultimate source of energy for life on earth. Cannabis likes as much direct sunlight as it can get, so try to choose a location that gets as much sunlight throughout the day as possible.

Do you have a spot in your house to set up or build a place to grow some plants?

Make sure that you have the proper amount of space to either start your plants early before moving them outdoors or grow them to maturity. If you are planning to have your plants indoors for a short amount of time, such as 4–6 weeks, you will only need enough space to fit the pots that you place under your grow light. But if you are planning to go through the vegetative and flowering stage indoors under lights, you will need to plan for more space, with a minimum of 12 x 12 inches (30 x 30 cm) per plant. The larger your plants grow, the more space they will need.

You can choose from a few options when looking for a space to set up a grow room for raising plants exclusively indoors. When at all possible, it is best to have a grow room that is contained either in a separate room or away from your everyday living space. A vacant room can be one of your best options, or you can use a basement. Grow tents (see page 50) are a good option for people who do not have a lot of extra space in their homes. If you have the space and skills, you can always build a small grow room in your home, basement, shop, or outbuilding on your property.

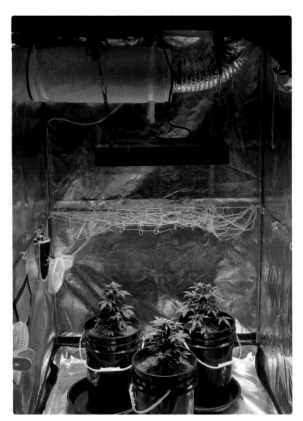

For indoor growers, a grow tent can transform any small space into an optimal growing environment. You can easily hook up a grow tent to lights, fans, timers, and other equipment. The reflective coating on the interior maximizes light intensity.

If you grow indoors, do you have electricity to run a light and some fans? Are the outlets on the same circuit breaker or different breakers?

When growing indoors, safety is of the utmost importance. If you are simply plugging in a low-wattage light, such as a fluorescent fixture or a small LED light, this is not much of a concern. But if you are setting up a full-scale grow room, consisting of powerful lights, exhaust and intake fans, timers, and more, it is *very* important that you make sure you are not overloading the breakers in your fuse panel. Fortunately, most breakers are designed to switch off the overloaded circuits before they get too hot, but you need to make sure that you do not try to draw more energy than they are designed to deliver. Check that you have the correct number of outlets and available power for the equipment that you want to run. I always recommend seeking the help of a qualified electrician during the planning process of setting up your room.

Can I keep my plants in a private space and safe from theft?

No matter where you decide to grow—whether it is indoors, outdoors, or a combination of the two—you should keep your cannabis away from sight and let as few people know about what you are doing as possible.

Even though cannabis is legal in many areas, the risk of theft is still very real, and the negative stigma that surrounds the plant is still all too common. The more people you tell about your garden, the greater your chances of someone mentioning it to a potential thief or anyone looking for a quick score or to create trouble for you by calling local authorities. There will always be people who are looking to take advantage of your hard work, including professional thieves who specialize in stealing cannabis. Although they generally target large grow operations, you do not want to attract their attention. For these reasons, try to grow your plants in a place that is the least visible to unscrupulous eyes (see page 44 for more information).

INDOOR VERSUS OUTDOOR GROWING

There are many factors to consider when deciding whether you will grow your cannabis indoors, outdoors, or a combination of the two. Most growers choose to grow either indoors or outdoors exclusively, but some do a combination of the two, starting their plants indoors for a few weeks to a month and then moving them outside to let the plants grow and mature with natural conditions under the sun. Other people may prefer to grow their plants entirely indoors, where every factor of the environment can be controlled and manipulated to deliver optimum results. There are benefits to each of these methods of growing cannabis. Find what method works for you using the information below, utilize the resources that you have available to you, and adapt to your environment.

Outdoor Growing

Growing cannabis outdoors is the way it has been done for thousands of years and is by far the most natural and environmentally friendly way to grow your plants. When at all possible, I recommend growing your cannabis plants outdoors in full sun. When planted in the ground and left to grow for the entire season, your plants are far more likely to reach their full genetic potential and develop more complex and diverse cannabinoid and terpene profiles. It is said that some of the best cannabis in the world is grown outside, under the sun in California. Its climate seems to be just about perfect for cannabis growing. For decades, the state has produced some of the finest flowers in the world. With that said, we can still grow amazing cannabis in many other regions around North America, and I know many people (including myself) who claim that the best cannabis they ever tried was grown outdoors, regardless of the area in which it was cultivated.

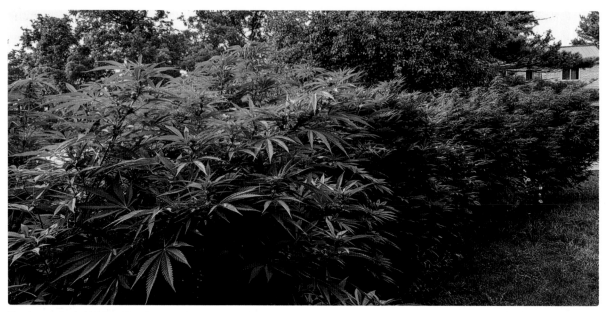

Planting your cannabis alongside other plants such as this heritage apple tree can keep them from the sight of nosy neighbors or thieves. Doing so will also increase the biodiversity of your garden and the health of your cannabis.

Pros:

- You let Mother Nature do a lot of the work. You can't beat the power of natural sunshine.

- Outdoor plants can grow much bigger and produce very large yields. NLD plants are especially more likely to grow to their full potential outdoors.

- Your costs will be lower as you are less dependent on the power grid. (Perhaps you might not be dependent on the power grid at all!)

- Many people believe that plants grown under the sun often have higher levels and a more diverse array of terpenes and cannabinoids. Contrary to what some people say and believe, the potency of the sun-grown cannabis can be the same as cannabis that has been grown indoors.

- You can camouflage your plants in gardens by surrounding them with other plants, such as trees, shrubs, and vines.

- Cannabis grows outdoors naturally. It is meant to thrive under the sun and in healthy, living, native soil. If you live in a northern climate, you will have fewer cultivars that you can grow, but you can always find success with autoflowers. The genetics of these varieties are getting better and better.

Cons:

- Bigger plants can require more maintenance and time to harvest, dry, cure, trim, and store because of their bigger yields.

- It may be harder to provide privacy and security for outdoor plants and keep thieves, wandering neighbors, and other visitors, such as guests, mail carriers, and delivery people from finding your patch. The plants' odor may also attract unwanted attention.

- Some cultivars will just not do as well grown outdoors, especially in northern climates. In northern climates, it can be hard (though nowhere near impossible) to grow top-quality flowers outdoors if you don't use autoflowers or early-finishing cultivars.

- Unless you are prepared and pick the best cultivars for your region, weather and environmental conditions can wreak havoc on your plants. Wind and rainstorms, drought, cold temperatures, and frost can all damage your crop.

Indoor Growing

Growing indoors began to become very popular in the 1980s and '90s, especially as lighting technology improved and led to larger yields. These yields often had higher potency that was made possible by maintaining optimal environmental conditions, artificial lighting, and hydroponic systems. (Hydroponic growing systems do not use soil, and the roots of the plants are suspended in a nutrient-rich water solution.) In a properly maintained environment, growers are able to get many harvests (sometimes six or more in one year) of trichome-laden buds.

By growing indoors, you can control the environmental conditions and keep your grow room at the optimum temperature and humidity. For many growers, having an indoor setup can be very rewarding and provide endless hours of gardening enjoyment throughout the year, which can be especially appealing to those who live in colder climates and are looking for a way to pass the time during the winter months.

Pros:

- You can control many aspects of the growing environment, such as its temperature, humidity, soil nutrients, air circulation, and ventilation.

- Indoor gardens are more secure from theft than outdoor gardens. You can also lock your grow room and keep guests from discovering it.

- You can produce very vibrant, colorful, high-potency plants. BLD plants, in particular, can grow well using many different indoor grow methods.

- Your plants can flower whenever you want, and you can have multiple harvests throughout a year, including during the winter.

- Indoor growing is ideal if you do not have a space to grow outdoors and can be a viable option for people who live in a northern climate.

Cons:

- It costs more money to set up, run, and maintain a grow room. You'll need to purchase equipment, such as grow lights, bulbs, and fans; perform maintenance on that equipment; and replace it as needed. Indoor grow rooms and high-intensity lights can also use a lot of electricity, which will lead to a higher-than-normal power bill.

- Indoor grows have a high environmental footprint because a lot of power is needed to run all the equipment required for a successful harvest. You also tend to use more material and equipment that eventually has to be thrown out once it has reached the end of its life span and is no longer functioning properly. Old lights, plastic to cover walls, fans, ductwork, and more will find their way to the landfill.

- A grow room can take up a lot of your time. For example, you need to constantly monitor and maintain the conditions in your grow room, create a regular watering schedule, and constantly be on the lookout for signs of pests and potential disease.

- There is a risk of fire. Though this risk is quite low, you must always make sure that you are not overloading your circuit breakers and have enough power to run your equipment safely. Safety is always paramount!

- Odor can be an issue when growing indoors. Without tools such as carbon filters, the smell of your plants might spread throughout your home.

- Pests and disease can easily run rampant in indoor growing operations and spoil an entire harvest quickly.

A Hybrid Approach

Cannabis growers can take a hybrid approach, growing your cannabis plants using both indoor and outdoor techniques. We will talk about three common hybrid approaches and when these options may make sense for you to employ.

Starting Indoors Then Moving Outdoors

If you live in a northern climate, it often makes the most sense to start your seeds or clones indoors under lights about 4–6 weeks before it is safe to move your plants outside. (You can keep them inside longer or shorter than this, if you like.) Starting your plants inside will give them time to gain strength before you harden them off to outdoor conditions (see page 121) and take them outside to face the elements. In many cases, this head start is all that your plants will need to adapt to a spring season in a northern climate and have enough time to grow into very large plants with significant yields.

Growing in Pots on a Deck or Balcony

If you do not have any garden space or you have nosy neighbors, you can keep your plants in pots. This approach can work out well for folks who live in towns, cities, or apartments with balconies. Although the plants will not grow as big as they would if they were planted in the ground, they will reach a decent size and produce a nice yield if they are planted in the proper-size pot and kept adequately watered throughout their life cycle.

Another benefit of growing your plants in this way is that you can bring your plant inside when the nights are cold and then put it back out in the morning. This can help you to extend your growing season by allowing you to avoid some of the cool spring nights as well as the potentially wet, cold, and frosty weather that comes to most areas during the fall. I have seen and grown some

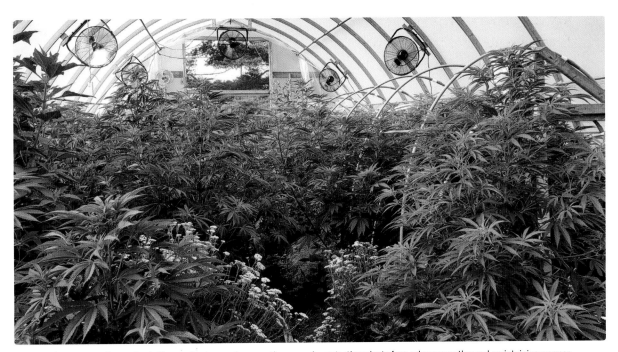

This greenhouse on our farm extends the growing season by a month or more by protecting plants from adverse weather and maintaining warmer temperatures. It is crucial to have proper ventilation and air circulation in a greenhouse to prevent disease. We control airflow by using exhaust and circulation fans and by rolling up the walls of the greenhouse.

beautiful plants over the years using this method, and some of them were located deep in the heart of large cities.

Hoop Houses and Greenhouses

Hoop houses and greenhouses are the ultimate hybrid approach, and they can produce some stellar results in terms of yield, quality, and potency of the flowers they produce. Greenhouses are contained areas, covered in either plastic or glass. They have the ability to ventilate air through a combination of exhaust fans and circulating fans and use electricity to run this equipment. Many of the professional greenhouses that are manufactured and used today can create conditions very similar to those in indoor grow rooms, but you can use the power of the sun and get by without any supplemental lighting.

A more low-key and low-tech option for the home grower is to build a hoop house by simply covering a series of hoops made from steel, PVC, or even wood with plastic sheets. Using plastic designed for greenhouses is the best, and most come with a UV protectant that will increase its life span. A hoop house will create an enhanced environment that protects your plants from some of nature's elements and traps heat inside the space, warming it well above the outside ambient air temperature.

Like pots and containers, hoop houses and greenhouses have the ability to lengthen the season for growers and give your plants a chance to grow earlier in the spring and longer in the fall. It is best to build these structures well before the growing season so that they are ready for your plants to move in. These shelters are often used with light deprivation techniques, whereby the structure is covered once a day by black tarps (or an automated shade cover) to supply less light to the plants (which creates a longer dark period). This triggers the plants to enter the flowering cycle. Some growers in places with warmer climates, such as California, can get three and sometimes even four harvests per season by employing these techniques. If you have the space and resources to buy or make a greenhouse or a hoop house, it can be a fun way to experiment with a number of different growing techniques.

FAQS & TROUBLESHOOTING

Q: How tall will my plants get?

A: That is a hard one to answer. There are a lot of factors that will affect the growth and overall height of your plant: genetics, growing style, nutrients, environmental conditions (such as amount of sun, rain, wind, storms, and more). Some plants will naturally get very tall (over 20 feet [6.1 m] with the right conditions), while others, such as many autoflowers, may max out at 2–4 feet (61 cm–120 cm). Do your research before committing to a specific cultivar. You can also learn about some techniques that can help you control height, if that is your objective. Generally speaking, your plants will most likely be somewhere between 4 and 10 feet (1.2 and 3 m) tall.

Q: How easily can I build a hoop house?

A: You can put together a hoop house quite easily. There are prefabricated greenhouse and hoop house kits that you can buy. You can build one with the materials and resources you have on hand. Check out some videos online, do some research, and you will find that there are many cost-effective ways to build a simple hoop house.

Q: What do I have to be concerned about if I decide to grow my plants in a greenhouse?

A: There are a number of things that you will want to be prepared for when growing in a greenhouse for the first time. The most important factors that will determine your success include having good air flow and ventilation, and the ability to control your temperature. Greenhouses can get very hot in the middle of the summer, and it may be worth investing in some equipment like fans or shutters to avoid high humidity and fluctuating temperatures, which can lead to mold and powdery mildew. There is a learning curve with growing in hoop houses and greenhouses, but do not let that hold you back. Build one, grow some plants in it, gain some experience, and dial in your systems!

Q: If I have the option to grow both indoors and outdoors, what would you recommend?

A: Both approaches will give you experience that will make you a better grower, but from the standpoint of regenerative agriculture, growing outside makes more sense. There are no energy costs, the plants get bigger, and you get to spend time outside. Outdoor growing uses far less energy and reduces the environmental impact of your garden. It's also easier on your wallet. Outdoor growing is the more natural way to go. Plants evolved growing under the sun and will reach and demonstrate their true potential in an outdoor environment. Plus, you will have many more opportunities to gain regenerative farming skills—closing loops, utilizing stacking functions, and letting your plants coexist with nature.

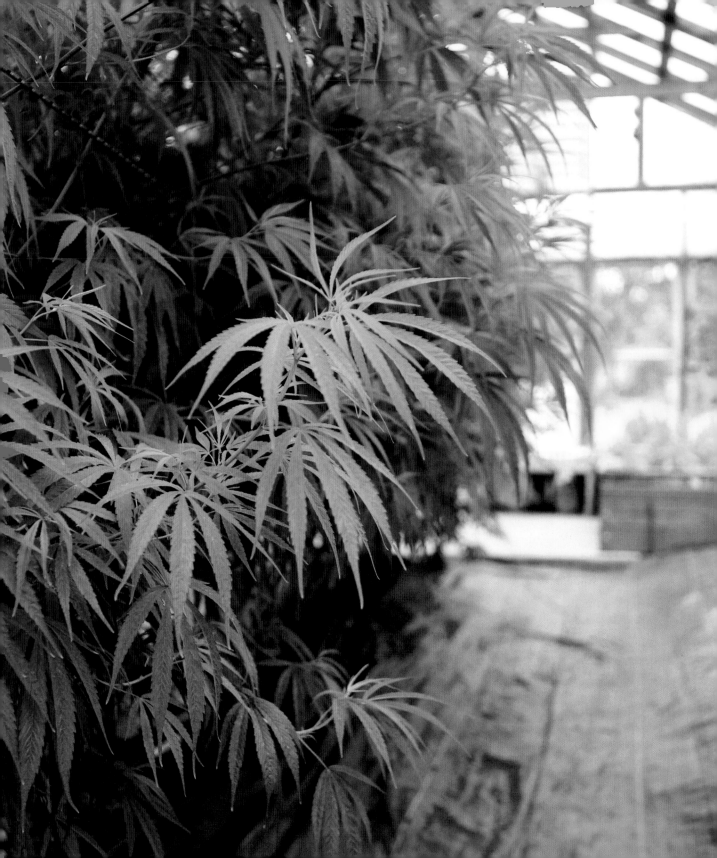

CHAPTER 4

< Setting Up Your Garden >

No matter where you are planning to grow your plants, it is important to have the right setup and maintain the proper environment for your plants to thrive. In this chapter, we are going to look at the key factors to think about when creating the optimum environmental conditions for your plants to thrive outdoors and indoors. For those of you who are new to growing, the information laid out in this chapter will lead to happy plants.

SETTING UP YOUR OUTDOOR GROW SPACE

There are a few things to consider when setting up your outdoor garden, and we will touch on many of them in the next couple of sections. As with most things related to growing cannabis, it is important to do your research, think through your ideas, and come up with a solid plan, especially before making any physical alterations to your landscape. Having a plan will save you time in the long run, allow you to use your energy more efficiently, as well as give you a reference to follow as you build your garden.

I encourage you to research as many organic gardening methods and techniques as possible and learn many different styles of outdoor gardening, especially ones that are practiced locally in your area. See "Resources" on page 233 for ideas if you are interested in taking a deeper dive into this subject. The more you learn, the more ideas and information you will have for working with your land and garden.

Choosing an Outdoor Space

Cannabis has the potential to be a very large plant, and you want to make sure you give it enough space to grow and thrive. The average height of cannabis is 4–10 feet (1.2–3 m), with some varieties reaching 20 feet (6.1 m), and they are about half as wide as their height. It is ideal to space each plant about 8–10 feet (2.4–3 m) apart, measuring from the center of the hole to the center of the next hole.

LEFT Cannabis grows in a greenhouse built in a private backyard.

< 43 >

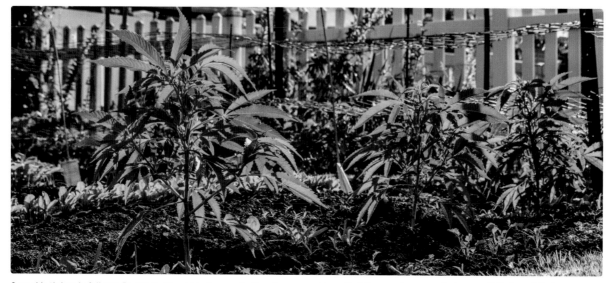

Cannabis thrives in full sun. Be sure to allow enough space for them to grow, and know that they may become quite large and block sunlight from reaching other plants in your garden.

If you do not have the room required for this amount of spacing, there is no need to worry. You have the option to plant your plants closer together. I have grown many plants over the years that were only 4–6 feet (1.2–1.8 m) apart and sometimes even closer.

Cannabis will soak up and photosynthesize as much light as you can give it, so look for an area that is in full sun for much of the day. It should receive a minimum of 6 hours of direct sunlight a day—the more the better.

If possible, try to pick an area where it is easy to hide your cannabis plants from the view of passersby and neighbors. You can do that by planting your cannabis out of view or even growing other large plants, such as elecampane, artichokes, and marshmallow, near and around your cannabis plants so that they do not stand out as much. Climbing vines, such as hops, peas, and morning glories, and small shrubs and trees in the background will also help your cannabis blend into the landscape a little more. Keep your yard and the space around your house well maintained so you do not draw any unwanted attention. You should also think about some potential security measures or deterrents that may thwart thieves. A simple motion detector light or a rope with cans and other noise-making objects can go a long way. Take privacy and security seriously—the last thing you want is someone to steal your prized plants just as you are getting ready to harvest and reap the rewards of your hard work. Depending on your area, these measures are not always necessary, but they definitely were essential in the past and will continue to be in some areas into the future. It is up to you to decide how discreet you need to be.

NO-TILL GARDENING

If at all possible, try to practice no-till methods in your garden. No-till gardening means that you do not turn and cultivate the soil each year before you begin planting. This method of gardening will help to improve the soil structure, limit compaction, prevent erosion, while helping the soil retain more water and nutrients. By avoiding tilling, you will build healthy living soil full of beneficial microbes and fungi, which will in turn support strong, healthy, and nutritious plants.

To get started, you will need to make sure that you are weeding your garden consistently and not letting undesirable plants go to seed. It is very helpful to add compost or manure to the top of the soil in the spring and then a layer of mulch about 8–12 inches (20–30 cm) thick. You can also do this in the fall as well when you close your garden down for the season. This layer of mulch will help to suppress the weeds, and when the mulch breaks down, it adds a rich layer of organic matter to your soil that will provide a habitat for beneficial microbes, fungi, and other forms of life.

Growing Cannabis in an Existing Garden

Cannabis can be a great addition to an already established garden. There is something special about having this plant growing alongside your vegetables, herbs, and ornamental flowers. I also think cannabis is happiest when it's growing alongside other plants as well. For example, you can have some smaller plants, such as lettuce, radishes, potatoes, carrots, smaller herbs, and flowers, growing underneath a cannabis plant.

Keep in mind that your cannabis will most likely be the tallest plants in the garden. You may want to put them on the north side of the garden so the plants get full southern exposure and avoid blocking off the light from the plants located behind them.

If you want to keep your cannabis out of sight, make it blend into your existing garden. That may mean growing plants in scattered locations around your garden or devoting a small row or section for your cannabis plants.

Companion Planting

I'm a big fan of polyculture—the practice of growing many species together. Why create separate gardens when we can have our food, medicine, and cannabis all growing together? Creating polyculture gardens that are rich in biodiversity is not only important for your plants, but also to the many beneficial insects, pollinators, and other wildlife that live in your area.

One way to build a polyculture garden is to practice companion planting. With companion planting, you'll look for plants that have a beneficial impact on one another throughout the growing season. Some plants, such as stinging nettle, may increase the potency of other plants that grow around it. Many pollinator-friendly plants may draw beneficial insects or repel pests. Others may nourish the soil and, in turn, the other plants that grow nearby. There are even plants that boost the oil and resin content of your cannabis plants and help them produce denser flowers and heavier yields.

In this section, you'll find lists of plants that do well with cannabis. The plants are grouped into different categories based on their benefits.

Companion Plants That Boost Growth

Alfalfa: A member of the legume family, alfalfa fixes nitrogen from the air into the soil via root nodules where *Rhizobium* bacteria reside. This helps to rebuild and replenish your soil and has been used for many years as a compost accelerant. A tea made from alfalfa is loaded with vitamins and minerals. You can apply the tea as a foliar spray (see page 68) or a soil drench (see page 205). Alfalfa is also a great source of mulch for your garden and will release nutrients into your soil as it gets rained on and decomposes.

Chamomile: Chamomile increases the resin production of cannabis and has been said to increase turgor in plants growing close to it. (Turgor is what makes living plant tissue rigid. Loss of turgor, resulting from the loss of water from plant cells, causes flowers and leaves to wilt.)

Comfrey: Comfrey can add fertility to your soil and a big boost of macro- and micronutrients to your garden. You can make it into a tea or use the "chop and drop" method—chopping the plant down and leaving the foliage to decompose in your garden. This method adds nutrients back into your soil and can act like a layer of mulch as well. Comfrey is very resilient and will grow back in no time.

Coriander: Coriander's blossoms will draw beneficial insects, such as parasitoid wasps and hoverflies. The scent of the plant may deter some insects from the garden as well. The seeds can be crushed and brewed into a tea and sprayed onto your plants as a natural insecticide to control spider mites and other pests. Coriander also helps to ward off aphids and potato beetles.

Valerian: Valerian is a good compost stimulant, helping with the assimilation of phosphorus into the soil. It is also used in some biodynamic preparations that can be sprayed onto your plants to protect them from frost in both the spring and fall.

Companion Plants That Repel Insects

Calendula: Calendula should be in every gardener's companion planting tool kit. It stimulates growth in neighboring plants and releases an insect-repelling chemical into the

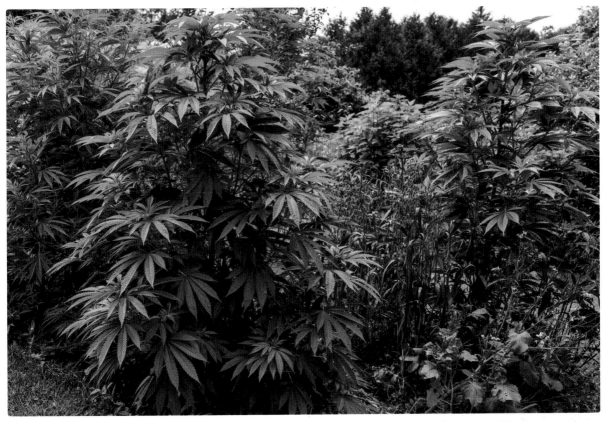

In this part of my garden, I planted cannabis alongside milk thistle, marshmallow, elecampane, Jerusalem artichokes, yarrow, echinacea, wormwood, valerian, strawflower, and a number of vegetables.

soil that helps deter root-feeding nematodes. The striking orange flowers attract beneficial nectar-eating insects and repel beetles, leafhoppers, and whiteflies. They can also lure aphids away from your cannabis while attracting beneficial insects, including hoverflies, lacewings, and ladybirds, which prey on aphids.

Coriander: Coriander is great at repelling potato beetles, aphids, and spider mites. They also help to attract hoverflies, tachinid flies, and a number of parasitoid wasps.

Dill: Dill attracts beneficial insects, such as hoverflies and honeybees, and ichneumonids and other parasitoid wasps. Spider mites are thoroughly repelled by dill, and it is also an effective repellent for aphids, cabbage looper, and squash bugs.

Peppermint: Peppermint is a versatile plant that will attract beneficial insects, such as bees, and can help repel aphids, ants, flea beetles, and mice. It is also an aggressive plant and will spread throughout your garden if it finds the conditions to be favorable.

Wormwood: Wormwood is a very strong-smelling plant that will deter aphids and flea beetles from neighboring plants. The small, yellow flowers attract ladybirds, lacewings, and hoverflies, which will prey on aphids.

Yarrow: Yarrow repels a number of bugs and attracts many beneficial predatory insects like aphid lions (which are lacewing larvae), ladybugs, and hoverflies, as well as several species of desirable parasitoid wasps. It is best planted on the edge of your gardens, as it can easily spread and begin to take over your bed.

Companion Plants That Improve Soil Health

Alfalfa: Alfalfa fixes nitrogen from the air into the soil and accumulates iron, magnesium, potassium and phosphorus into its plant tissue. It grows rather quickly and is a good plant for the "chop-and-drop" technique (chop it and leave it on the soil surface as a mulch). The deep roots help break up the soil, which, in turn, increases water penetration and retention and slows down the evaporation process.

***Cerastium* spp.:** Working well as living mulch, they grow quickly and provide shade to the soil. They also help retain water in the soil and actually increase water penetration. You can cut them back a number of times over the growing season and let them decompose on top of the soil.

Chamomile: Chamomile will accumulate calcium, potassium, and sulfur in its foliage and then release it back into the top layer of soil after the plants die back.

Daikon radishes: These vegetables help to aerate the soil and create pathways for oxygen and water. They can grow quite deep. Plant them in the spring or fall to give them time to get established. You can either harvest them or let them rot in place.

White and red clover: Both members of the legume family, these plants fix nitrogen into the soil. They can also be used as a living mulch that helps retain water in the soil They attract small pollinators and can provide cover to the soil for a couple of seasons or more (depending on whether you let them go to seed).

Other Plants to Consider Growing

Chives and onions: It is said that chives and onions can improve the flavor of plants growing around them, and they can also help to repel various pests, including aphids. They take up little space and can be planted under and around the canopy of your cannabis plants.

Elecampane: This tall member of the *Asteraceae* family has a sunflower-like flower and works well to shade the soil and prevent weeds from encroaching into your gardens. It attracts many insects and is a great medicinal herb for the lungs and the immune system. These plants create a lot of biomass in the garden and will help you to build soil year after year.

Marshmallow: Marshmallow is a beautiful plant that will attract pollinators to your garden as well as create shade with its tall flower spikes. It has been used as a medicinal herb for centuries and will flower profusely beginning in midsummer. It also creates a fair amount of biomass, which can be added to your compost.

Sweet alyssum: This plant makes an excellent cover crop or living mulch, blooms extensively, and is great at attracting beneficial insects, such as many small parasitoid wasp species whose larvae will feed on aphids, caterpillars, and other pests.

Tobacco: Tobacco is a large plant that can be used as a natural insecticide when made into a tea and used as a spray. It also attracts many butterflies, moths, and hummingbirds to the garden.

Vegetables: Many common vegetables do well with cannabis, including potatoes, carrots, lettuce, onions, garlic, Swiss chard, and kale, to name just a few. I encourage you to experiment with mixing many different food plants into your cannabis gardens.

SETTING UP AN INDOOR GROW SPACE

This book is designed to teach you how to grow your plants outdoors, but we will cover how to set up an indoor growing space as well. Although it does not delve into every detail related to indoor growing, it will help you set up a grow space that will meet your plants' basic requirements.

Choosing a Space

When planning your indoor grow space, the first thing to think about is the number of plants you are planning to grow, how long you want to grow them for, and how big you want them to be when you harvest them. This will help you determine the amount of space that you need. The longer you leave your plants in the vegetative stage, the bigger they will get. Small plants that are 12–16 inches (30–40 cm) tall may only need 3–4 inches (7.5–10 cm) between them, while taller plants may need a foot or more. If your plants are too tightly packed together, there will not be enough airflow, and they will be more susceptible to pest and disease.

Next, consider where you can set up a grow space in your house. Is there a place in your house that is not being used and can be turned into a grow room? Is there a spot in your basement where you could create a grow space or put a grow tent? If you do not need a lot of space or are only growing a few plants, you may be able to get away with using a corner of a room, a closet, or setting up a light next to a south-facing window, which will provide extra sunlight throughout the day. A solarium or sunroom can work great for a small number of plants as well.

It is best to pick a space where the temperature and humidity do not change drastically over the course of the day or between daytime and nighttime. The steadier the temperature and humidity, the better. Places such as unheated sheds and outbuildings will generally not work well without an external heat source and constant monitoring. It is easier to work with a basement that is slightly too cool or a room in a house, rather than a space that is not ideal and requires constant monitoring because of fluctuating temperature and humidity levels. Your chosen area should have a power source, with an outlet or two for plugging in your lights, timers, and fans.

There are always workarounds and modifications you can make if your space is not ideal. For example, if your area gets too cold at night, you can set up a small heater with a thermostat that will regulate the nighttime temperature and keep it at an optimum level. If your space gets too humid, you can use a dehumidifier; conversely, you can use a humidifier that will put additional moisture into the air if you live in a dry climate.

Grow Tents

For many people, grow tents can be a great option if you have limited space or do not have a room in your house that you can dedicate to growing cannabis. However, they are a little pricey. They come in various sizes and are lined with a reflective material with holes that allow for exhaust and intake vents. If you have an open, unfinished basement or would like to keep everything contained without having to build a separate room, these tents can be a convenient choice. You can also buy full kits that come with lights, fans, timers, and filters. They are a good choice for many growers, but they might not be for everyone. Do your research and make your decisions based on your specific needs, environment, and conditions.

Lighting

When growing cannabis inside, you will need some form of artificial lighting. Many people try to start their seeds on a sunny windowsill. Although this may work if you have a large south-facing

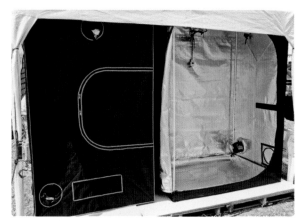

A grow tent can be used in small spaces and offers an alternative to building or adapting an entire room in your home for your plants.

window, it is not an ideal situation. Most windows do not get enough direct sunlight for your plants to thrive, especially during the flowering stage.

Always keep in mind that the more lights you use, the more power you will also use. Many lights, such as high-intensity discharge (HID) ones, also produce a lot of heat. You can either use this heat to warm your room, especially in the winter months, or vent it out of your room to maintain a steady temperature and humidity. If your room overheats in the hotter summer months, it could have devastating results.

When your plants are growing in the vegetative stage, you will want to turn your lights on for 18 hours and turn them off for 6 hours during each 24-hour period. When you are ready to transition your plants into the flowering stage, you will need to give your plants 12 hours of light and 12 hours of darkness (more on this in chapter 9, page 153). The light period is when the lights in your grow space are on. The dark period is when your lights are off.

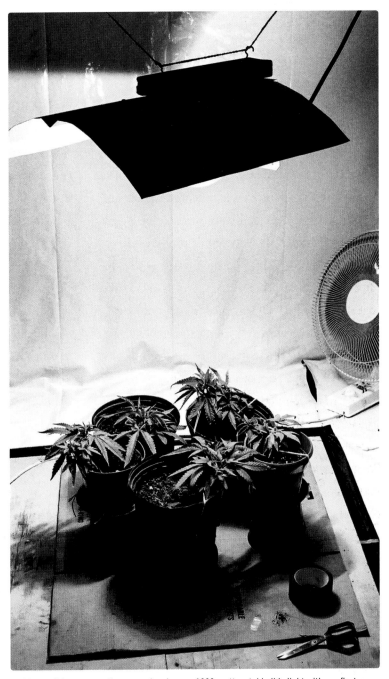

In this small home grow, the grower has hung a 1000-watt metal halide light with a reflector. The walls are covered in a reflective white plastic, and an oscillating fan moves air around the space. A simple setup like this may be all you need to start growing cannabis at home.

To give your plants the right amount of light efficiently, you will need to set your lights up with an automatic timer. (Trust me, you will not be anywhere near as efficient and reliable as a timer!) Your lights should be hung from the ceiling so they are directly above your plants. There will be different requirements for the amount of space needed between the light and the canopy of your plants. It is very important to follow the recommendation provided by the manufacturer of the light that you are using so that you do not accidentally burn your plants.

Here you will find descriptions of some lighting options. You can choose the one that best suits your needs, space, and budget. Get the best lights you can afford, and invest in better ones if you know you are going to want to keep growing long into the future.

If you are just going to start your seeds indoors 4–6 weeks before moving them outdoors, you may be fine using fluorescent lights. (Do not use incandescent lights, as they do not give off enough light and will result in weak, spindly plants.) But if you are planning to grow bigger plants, illuminate a large space, or have your plants flower indoors, you will want to look at some more powerful light options, such as LED (light-emitting diode) or HID (high-intensity discharge) lights. If you're unsure or just starting out, it is always a good idea to visit your local grow or lighting store and speak with an expert.

Fluorescents and Compact Fluorescent Lights

Fluorescent lights and compact fluorescent lights (CFLs) are probably your cheapest and most cost-effective option. You may even have some lying around your house right now, and they can easily be purchased at your local hardware, big-box, or grow store. They do not produce much heat and can be kept close to the plants, a benefit if your space is small.

If you use fluorescent lights, you can look for the thinner, newer T5 models or the larger, older T8s and T12s. If you have an old two-bulb fluorescent light fixture and are buying new bulbs for it, try to purchase one that is "cool white" and a "warm" one. They will be labeled on the packaging. There are also newer bulbs that are specifically designed for growing, but they will be more expensive.

Though fluorescent lights and CFLs work fine for growing seedlings and young plants, they are not strong enough to produce top-quality, dense flowers.

Light-Emitting Diodes

Light-emitting diodes (LEDs) have come a long way in a fairly short time. The technology has advanced to the point where it is a very viable choice for growing cannabis in both the vegetative and flowering cycles. They are very efficient and do not produce the heat that HID lighting does. These lights also use a lot less electricity, which can result in large cost savings on your power bill.

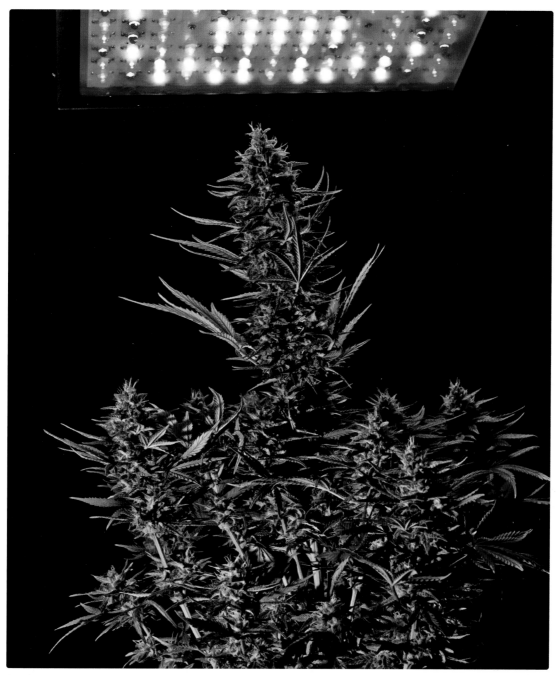

This style of LED light emits a mixture of red and blue light. For adult plants grown completely indoors, you may want to purchase a broad-spectrum LED light that incorporates more "white" light, which will emit a wider range of wavelengths that works for all stages of growth and increases quality and yields.

They are expensive, especially the good ones, and there are many lights on the market that are cheaply made and do not deliver on their promises. Do your homework and spend the money to make sure you get a quality product. The lifetime of high-quality LEDs and the savings they give you in electricity costs can help you recoup the extra upfront cost of purchasing the lights quite quickly.

High-Intensity Discharge

High-intensity discharge (HID) lighting is what most old-school growers have been using for decades. They are incredibly bright, creating a high amount of lumens, which measure how much light you are getting from a bulb, and emitting a broad spectrum of light. These lights come in a few different types, including metal halide (MH), high-pressure sodium (HPS), and the newer ceramic metal halide (CMH).

MH and HPS lights generally come in 400, 600, and 1,000 watts and are often sold in packages that contain a ballast, a bulb, a socket, and a reflector. Many new digital ballasts will let you use both metal halide and HPS bulbs in the same unit by simply flipping a switch, allowing the home grower to only purchase one ballast, socket, and reflector to cover both the vegetative and flowering cycles. (A ballast regulates the current being delivered to the bulbs and ensures that there is sufficient voltage to start the bulbs.)

CMH lights are more efficient and a newer development. They generally use less power and create a little less heat than HPS and MH. You can purchase one bulb for vegetative growth and one bulb for flowering and use them in the same ballast.

These lights are known to produce some of the nicest buds in an indoor environment, though LEDs are quickly catching up. HID lights come in many different wattages, varying from 150 watts to the best-known 1,000 watts. Many growers have used the higher "blue" light of the MH for vegetative growth and the higher "red" light of the HPS for flowering. Although there are conversion ballasts that run both lights, you will need to invest in separate bulbs if you're using MH and HPS. Many new digital ballasts will even allow you to run the light at a lower wattage (600 watts, 750 watts, and 1,000 watts).

> **TIP:** To cut down on electricity costs, it is often cheaper to run your lights at night when electricity is commonly charged at a discounted rate. This can also help add heat to your grow space during the cooler months and allow you to use less electricity to run heaters.

MEASURING WAVELENGTHS AND LUMENS

Light can be measured in many ways, and it is important to understand that plants do not "see" or experience light in the same way that we do. Light is made up of many separate bands of colors, and each color in the spectrum supports and encourages a different type of growth. Blue light encourages stem and leaf growth, white or neutral light promotes normal to rapid growth, while red light promotes flowering. Although plants use many of the colors of the light spectrum, red and blue are the most important and promote photosynthesis most effectively. Lights that are specifically designed for growing will have information about the spectrum it emits along with a diagram on the box.

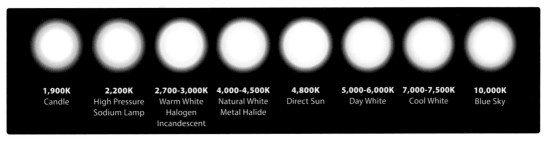

| 1,900K | 2,200K | 2,700-3,000K | 4,000-4,500K | 4,800K | 5,000-6,000K | 7,000-7,500K | 10,000K |
| Candle | High Pressure Sodium Lamp | Warm White Halogen Incandescent | Natural White Metal Halide | Direct Sun | Day White | Cool White | Blue Sky |

Color temperature, which is used to describe the color of lights, is measured in Kelvins. Lights with low color temperatures are warm, whereas lights with high color temperatures are cool.

In addition to considering the wavelengths, you'll need to consider how many lumens you'll require to light your space. The number of lumens depends on the square footage. You can use the chart below to match up the proper HID light that you would need to illuminate your grow space.

LUMENS PROVIDED BY HID LIGHTS

Wattage	Area	Lumens
250	2 x 2 feet	25,000
400	3 x 3 feet	45,000
600	3½ x 3½ feet	60,000
1,000	5 x 5 feet	100,000

NOTE: You can use this chart for LED lights as well. Most LED lights will include comparisons to HID lights, which were the standard in the industry for many years.

Maintaining the Proper Environment

When growing indoors, it is very important to maintain the proper growing environment. You need to control the temperature, humidity, fresh air coming into your room (intake), and "old" air being vented out of your room (exhaust). Doing so will make a difference in the health and vitality of your plants and your ability to produce a successful harvest of top-shelf buds. The good news is that it can be done quite easily with a little know-how and the proper equipment.

Timers

Automating your grow space with the use of various timers can cut down on the time you need to spend turning equipment on and off. It will also help you to maintain the proper growing conditions in your room both day and night.

Perhaps the most important function of a timer is to turn your lights on and off on a set daily schedule. Make sure that this is consistent each and every day; the easiest way to do this is with a plug-in wall timer. You can find these at your local hardware, big-box, or grow store. Just be sure that they are rated to handle the wattage and amperage of the lights you are using. If you have multiple lights plugged into one outlet, you may want to find a timer that is made to handle this extra power. These advanced timers can be expensive, but they are not something that you should skimp on. The last thing you want in your grow space is a fire hazard.

You can put other equipment on a timer as well, including dehumidifiers, heaters, oscillating fans, and exhaust and intake fans. There are also more advanced timers with built-in thermostats that allow you to pick your settings and heat or cool your room as needed. These days, there are even units that can deliver all the vital information about the conditions in your grow space directly to your smartphone (though that may be more than you need at this point).

Temperature

Be sure you maintain a steady temperature and avoid any wild fluctuations in your grow space. Inconsistent temperatures can make your plants susceptible to powdery mildew, mold, pests, and more (see chapter 13).

The ideal temperature for your grow space is between 72°F and 76°F (22°C and 24.5°C). At night, the temperature can be a little cooler, but be sure that it does not drop more than 5°F–10°F (2°C–5°C). If the temperature is too cold at night (15°F [8°C] or colder), you will reach the dew point, meaning that moisture will began to settle on your plants. This excess humidity can increase the likelihood of mold and powdery mildew forming. Temperatures in excess of 85°F (29°C) or below 55°F (13°C) will slow or potentially stop growth, preventing your plants from thriving.

It's important to have at least one thermometer in your grow room that records the minimum and maximum temperature each day. This way, you can check what the lowest temperature was during the plant's dark period and what the highest temperature was during its light period. This data will make it easier not only to maintain the optimal temperature, but also to diagnose problems that may arise. It is best to have the sensor of these thermometers located near the canopy of your plants or just below them.

Depending on the conditions inside your grow space, you may need to invest in a small portable heater to maintain a warm enough temperature during the dark period, especially in the winter months. (Oil-filled radiant heaters work well for this.) In the summer months, you may need to invest in an air conditioner to cool down your room. Another way to potentially heat and cool your room is by using your exhaust and air-intake fans through ventilation (more on this on page 60).

Humidity

Maintaining a humidity level of between 50 and 60 percent during the vegetative stage and 40 and 50 percent during the flowering stage will help to keep your plants healthy and happy. It is best to keep your humidity as stable as possible, especially when transitioning between dark and light periods in your grow space. When your humidity is too high, there is an excess of water vapor in the air, providing ideal conditions for mold to thrive.

Since most spaces will tend to be on the humid side, a dehumidifier that allows you to maintain a specific humidity level is a great investment. If you live in an arid place, you may want to consider picking up a humidifier instead to put moisture into the air. But be careful. Humidifiers often work too well and can lead to problems if not properly monitored.

There are many other ways you can control the humidity in your grow space. For instance:

- Raising the temperature will generally increase humidity in your room. Increasing the amount of cool air supplied to your grow space will decrease humidity.

- You can place a bucket of water in your room, which will evaporate into the air, causing humidity to slightly increase (essentially a primitive "humidifier").

- Make sure your grow space is properly sealed to avoid changes in humidity levels.

- Use intake and exhaust fans to remove or add moist or dry air into your grow space.

Regardless of where you live, it is very important to have a hygrometer, ideally one that is combined with a thermometer that records minimum and maximum readings. This very valuable and inexpensive tool can be a game changer when diagnosing environmental issues in your grow space.

RECOMMENDED GROW ROOM CONDITIONS

Growing Stage	Lighting	Temperature
Seedling/Cloning	Light Period: 18 hours Dark Period: 6 hours Fluorescents, CFLs, low-wattage LEDs, and other low-intensity lights work best.	75–85°F (24–29°C) as seeds are sprouting and clones are rooting; decrease to 72–76°F (22–24°C) as seedlings and clones continue growing Using a heat mat under your tray of seedlings or clones will raise the temperature a few degrees higher than the ambient air temperature.
Vegetative	Light period: 18 hours Dark period: 6 hours Use HID or LED lights. If using HID lights, metal halide lights are best.	72–76°F (22–24°C)
Flowering	Light period: 12 hours Dark period: 12 hours Use HID or LED lights. If using HID lights, high-pressure sodium lights are best.	72–76°F (22–24°C) You can allow the nights to get colder near the end of flowering stage: 65–70°F (18–21°C).

Humidity Level	Special Needs	Tips
70–80% or higher as seeds are sprouting and clones are rooting; decrease to 50–60% as seedlings and clones continue growing For clones that are rooting, increase the humidity to 100% for the first couple days; decrease it to 90% for the next 5 days; and decrease it again to 75–80% the following week until you see signs of roots. If your plants start to wilt, increase the humidity.	Seeds do not need light until they sprout and break the surface of the soil, but clones need to be put under lights right away.	If using humidity domes to root your clones, be sure to take the lid off for 1 minute per day to exchange the air inside.
50–60%	Make sure your plants have an adequate amount of nitrogen for optimal vegetative growth.	Look up the Vapor Pressure Deficit (VPD) chart online, and you can find out which combinations of temperature and humidity levels are optimal for cannabis growth.
40–50%	Make sure your plants have adequate amounts of phosphorus and potassium for the flowering stage.	Be sure not to overwater your plants during this stage (as they will need less water), and maintain a lower humidity in your grow space.

Air Circulation

Maintaining airflow over and under the leaves of your cannabis plants is important. This helps to keep your plants healthy and thriving. You want to make sure that the air does not sit and become stale. You can ensure that air is moving and circulating throughout your grow space by using oscillating fans that you can get at your local hardware or grow store. They come in a variety of shapes, sizes, and strengths. Some will sit on the floor, others can be mounted on the wall, still others will clip onto something stationary in your room. You want to have your plants gently moving in the wind of the fan, but be careful not to blast air directly at a plant to avoid overpowering it and stunting its growth.

Ventilation

For indoor grow spaces, it is very important to ventilate your grow area. Proper ventilation will remove hot, humid, oxygen-rich air out of your grow space, while bringing cool, carbon-dioxide-rich air in. This is especially crucial if you are using a grow tent or a well-sealed room as your growing environment. If the smell of cannabis (especially during flowering) is a concern, you can connect charcoal or carbon filters to your exhaust fan.

When setting up an exhaust fan, it is best to mount it near the ceiling (where the warmest air is) and place your intake fan or vent near the floor or midway up the wall. Make sure that your intake fan is either the same size as or slightly smaller than your exhaust fan. This creates "negative" pressure, ensuring that you are drawing in fresh air without allowing odors to escape your room. These fans can pull air out of a room much more efficiently than they can push air out, so be sure to install an air vent or intake fan that allows fresh air to enter your grow room as the old air exits.

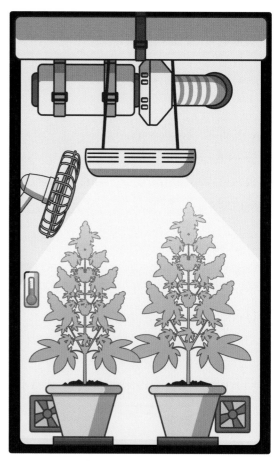

It is ideal for intake fans to be placed near the floor or halfway up the wall, whereas exhaust fans should be arranged at the top of your indoor grow space. This arrangement will ventilate your grow space most efficiently.

CALCULATING AIR EXCHANGE

You will want to have a fan that can completely remove and replenish the air in your grow room once every two minutes (or once per minute, if you are having issues with too much heat). The amount of air that inline fans can pull out is measured in cubic feet per minute (CFM).

To measure the volume of air in your room, use this equation:

$$\text{length of the room} \times \text{width of the room} \times \text{height of the room} = \text{total volume in cubic feet}$$

For example, if your grow room was 8 x 8 x 8 feet, then it would have a volume of 512 cubic feet. If you want to remove the air out of your room every two minutes, divide your volume by two. In this example, you would want a fan with a minimum of 256 CFM.

Safety

Safety should always be your number-one consideration when planning your grow space. You want your space to be set up in an organized, efficient, and safe way.

Make sure that you are not plugging too many devices into one outlet. Doing so can overwhelm your circuit breakers. For most of you, this should not be a problem. But if you decide to increase the number of lights or use heaters or dehumidifiers that draw more power, make sure that your power source can handle this electrical usage safely.

Always pay attention to how much power you are using. You do not want to overload your breakers. Most houses in North America have 15-, 20-, or 25-ampere breakers and a 120-volt circuit. To determine how many watts you can run, multiply the number of amperes that your breaker can handle with the voltage of your circuit. For example, if you have a 20-ampere breaker on a 120-volt circuit, you can technically run 2,400 watts on that circuit. However, I would recommend running less so that you are not close to the threshold for overloading the circuit; that is, only one 1,000-watt HID light per circuit. Take some time and do some research. Be sure to consult an electrician if you have any concerns or questions.

Make sure that all your plugs are completely plugged into the outlet at all times and that they are not generating heat. If they are hot to the touch, there is a problem that you need to investigate. You should get into a habit of checking all your power cords and outlets on a regular basis.

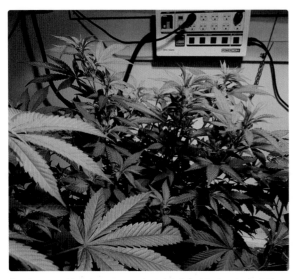
Growing cannabis indoors can require a lot of electrical equipment. There are some devices, such as the light controller shown in this photo, that will let you run multiple lights on one timer safely and efficiently.

Avoid overloading any outlet or circuits. If your breakers are constantly shutting off your power supply, try unplugging some of your equipment and make sure it is plugged into another circuit.

Store your cords properly, and always make sure your electrical outlets are mounted on a wall and kept up off the floor. Water and electricity do not mix. Make sure that your cords are kept off the ground, and avoid storing them in a place where they could come into contact with water or moist conditions. If you are using 1,000-watt lights, you also want to be aware of the heat that comes off your ballast, making sure that it, too, will not come into contact with moisture or water. It is always a good idea to either mount your ballasts to a wall or keep them off the ground using a couple of bricks or concrete blocks.

Keep your grow space off-limits to children, pets, and houseguests. I recommend having a lock on the door to your space or grow room. If you have children, it is best to have a talk with your children and let them know that this space is off-limits. For houseguests, you can put a sign on the door or near the grow area to indicate the same. It is best to keep pets away from this space as well. You do not want them entering this space as they could inadvertently knock something over or unplug a piece of your equipment. When at all possible, try your best to make your grow space child- and pet-proof, even if they do not have access to it.

Practice fire safety. Always have working smoke detectors in your grow space. Keep a fire extinguisher nearby and make sure it is kept in good working order. Clear away any flammable materials, including dried leaf and plant material, flammable liquids, trash, and debris, and store them outside your grow space. Keep your grow space clean and uncluttered at all times. A clean grow space is a happy and safe grow space. If you are concerned about fire, consider using LED lighting that draws less power and does not create the heat and high temperature that a HID lighting kit does.

Only use safety-approved equipment that is in good working order. Do not use old, damaged, or outdated lights, ballasts, timers, and extension cords. When it comes to anything involving electricity and lighting, never look for shortcuts!

Always wear protective eyeglasses when working in your grow space. There are eyeglasses that are specifically designed for LED and HID lighting. They will block out any harmful rays, such as UV light. Although sunglasses will protect your eyes, they will give you a discolored view of your plants, whereas grow glasses are designed to allow you to view your plants without interference, while also protecting your eyes.

FAQS & TROUBLESHOOTING

Q: Do I have to worry about companion plants taking over my garden? How do I make sure companion plants don't crowd out my cannabis plants?

A: When choosing companion plants, be sure to research how big they grow and what spacing is recommended for each plant. If they are encroaching on your cannabis plants, you can always prune them. When choosing your plants, find out if they are annuals, biennials, or perennials, and plant accordingly.

Q: Do I need to purchase expensive lights?

A: The answer depends on how you will use the lights. If you are just starting seeds and growing your seedlings under lights for a month or so before moving your plants outside, you do not need an expensive light. You can easily get by with some inexpensive lights, such as T5, T8, or T12 fluorescent lights. However, if you are going to try to flower your plants indoors, it is best to invest in a good light that will be more expensive in order to ensure a successful harvest.

Q: Is it really that important to pay attention to details like temperature or air circulation?

A: Yes, it is important to monitor all these details. Do you have to? No, but if you want to avoid potential issues, such as pests, disease, and unhealthy plants, it is best to do everything you can to maintain a proper and ideal environment for your plants.

Q: Will my plants be permanently harmed if the temperature and humidity levels are off for a short period?

A: No, as long as you catch the issue in time, your plants will regain their health. That said, if your temperature or humidity is off for a few days or more, you are a lot more likely to experience issues with slowed plant growth, pests, or disease, which can have a very detrimental effect on your plants. This is why it is best to monitor your grow space every day and use timers, thermometers, and hygrometers, as well as thermostats, to switch your equipment on and off automatically. There is a learning curve with indoor growing (just as there is with outdoor growing). Pay attention to your environmental conditions as well as the health of your plants, and you will gain many skills that will allow you to grow and maintain healthy plants.

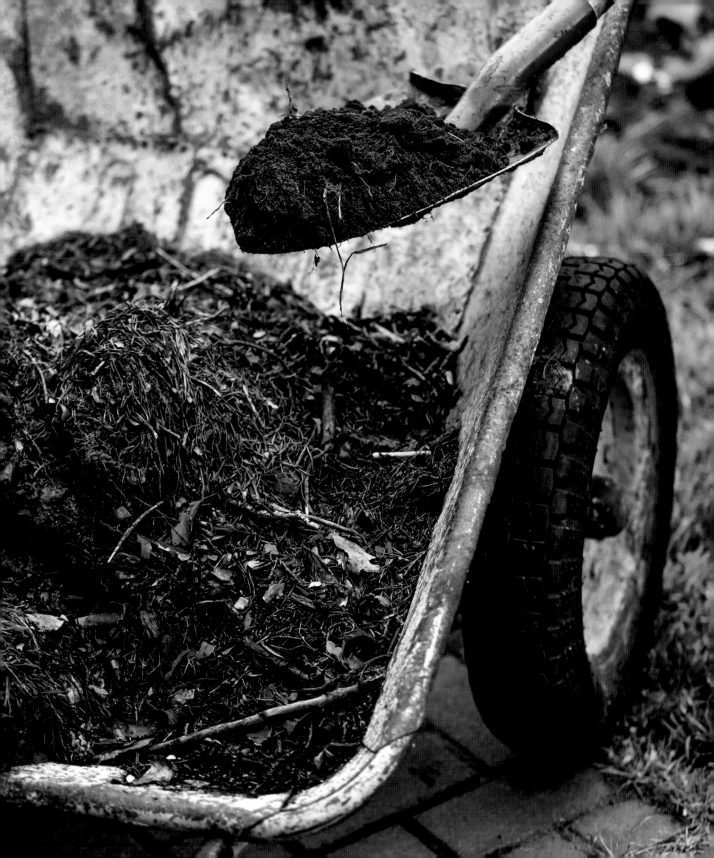

CHAPTER 5

< Soil & Nutrients >

When you nurture your soil, you give it life and vitality that is then transferred to your plants. In this chapter, we will cover how to build healthy soil that will provide all the nutrients that your plants will need and what to do if your soil is less than ideal. You'll find information about working with your native soil, using organic amendments that can be added to your soil to provide missing nutrients, techniques to build healthy living soil, and advice on using bottled nutrients.

SOIL REQUIREMENTS

Cannabis does best in a well-drained, noncompacted soil that is high in organic matter. The optimal pH of the soil is between 5.5 and 6.5. Whether you grow outdoors or indoors (or a hybrid of both), I encourage you to work with your native soil, whenever possible, and work toward regenerating the life and vitality within it. When growing indoors, it is always a good idea to incorporate some native soil into your mix.

When you're starting out, I recommend you have your soil tested. There is most likely a university or government agency in your area that can test your soil. In the United States, you can contact your local Natural Resources Conservation Service or extension office at the USDA Service Center for your county to learn about soil testing resources. If you live in Canada, there are a number of accredited soil-testing laboratories recommended by each province. You can find a list of these labs online. A soil test will tell you what nutrients and minerals are present in your soil and what may be lacking. This will help you decide whether you need to add soil amendments (see page 71), homemade fertilizers, or bottled

LEFT Compost is one of many amendments (see page 71) that can improve the health and vitality of your soil by supporting countless beneficial microbes and fungi in your garden's soil.

< 65 >

nutrients (see page 80) to your soil. If you do not want to go through the process of testing your soil, you can always plant your cannabis in the ground, observe how the plants grow, and make adjustments to the soil as needed.

PLANT NUTRITION

When people talk about plant nutrition and fertilizers, they often focus on macronutrients, especially nitrogen, phosphorus, and potassium (the N-P-K that you find on fertilizer labels stands for these three elements). Macronutrients are elements that plants require in relatively large amounts. Most soils contain high amounts of nitrogen, phosphorus, and potassium as well as other macronutrients, such as calcium, magnesium, sulfur, and carbon.

While macronutrients are impor-tant, your plants will also need micronutrients, trace minerals that they will use in smaller amounts. These are found in lower quantities in your soil and consist of elements such as iron, boron, copper, manganese, zinc, cobalt, chlorine, and molybdenum. Organic compost made using old plant stalks, hay and straw, deciduous leaves, and vegetables is rich in many micronutrients.

Your plant receives most of its nutrients through the soil. Though most soils contain a lot of the nutrients that your plants need, they may not be in a form that is bioavailable to them, meaning that your plants cannot absorb these nutrients. This is where the microbial life and fungal life in your soil come in.

Many people involved in regenerative agriculture often talk about "living soil." This term refers to soil full of microscopic organisms, including bacteria, fungi, and a plethora of other species. Living soil is truly alive with life, hence its name. These soil microbes are important because they feed on and break down organic matter, making the nutrients contained in this matter bioavailable to your plants. Fungal networks in the soil also help your plant's roots find and access those nutrients. It is through this symbiotic relationship between your plant and the microbes in your soil that your plants can achieve their full potential.

The microbes in your soil are also why synthetic fertilizers are not ideal. When nutrients come from a synthetic source or are overapplied, they can have a negative effect on the many

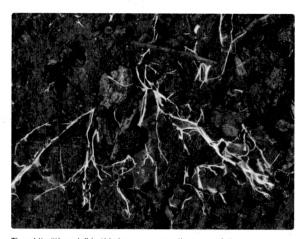

The white "threads" in this image are mycelium, one of the many beneficial fungi that live in soil. The presence of mycelium is a sign that your soil is in good health.

organisms that live in soil. Products derived from animal matter (such as bone and blood meal), manure, and plant matter (such as crop residues or compost) can provide macronutrients in a form that is readily available for your plants without those negative effects.

Your plants have a natural intelligence that can communicate with the life and nutrients in your soil and take up exactly what they need, when they need it. When your soil is alive and healthy, your plants will have nearly everything they need to grow—all you have to do is add water.

BUILDING LIVING SOILS

Building healthy living soils will go a long way toward providing a great environment for your cannabis plants to thrive. This process starts with your native soil. Whenever possible, use it as a base on which to build, adding organic matter, such as compost, manure, and mulch, to provide additional nutrients. There are other key soil-building principles that are important to practice, and many are covered in this book. You will learn about cover cropping (see page 192), no-till methods (see page 45), and ways to encourage the colonization and proliferation of beneficial microorganisms and healthy fungal networks in your soil.

Building living soils takes time and does not happen overnight, but by following some of the advice in this book, along with doing your own research on the subject, you will be well on your way to bringing life, health, and vitality back into your soil. There are many examples of people from around the world who have transformed land that has been abused and stripped of topsoil into a lush and vibrant space, teeming with life. Many modern and industrial agricultural practices, which include tilling the land, using synthetic fertilizers, and a whole host of chemical pesticides and herbicides, have come at a great cost, hurting the health of the world's soil and the life we share with other living creatures on this planet. Nurturing living soil offers another way forward, and it is up to us to make the changes, no matter how small, to swing the tide toward proper land stewardship and the regeneration of our soil.

If working with and building soil health is something you are interested in doing, I highly encourage you to venture down this path. It is very fulfilling to stand beside your garden that is bursting with life and healthy plants and know that the plants have all the nutrients they need. It will also allow you to avoid overpriced bottled nutrients (see page 80) and the need to feed your plants constantly.

FOLIAR FEEDING

Most nutrients are delivered to your plants through the soil. Foliar feeding offers an alternative method, using a water-based solution. Rather than adding the solution to the soil during watering, you spray it onto the aboveground parts of your plants. It is one of the quickest ways to deliver nutrients, which are absorbed directly into the vascular system through the leaves and stomata. Although not a substitute for healthy soil, foliar feeding is a quick and effective way to deliver nutrients to your plants, especially if they are suffering from a nutrient deficiency. It can also be used to treat stress, disease, and drought.

Cover your plants with a fine mist, but avoid leaving them dripping wet. Be sure to spray both the tops and bottoms of the leaves whenever possible. The best time to spray your plants is when the sun is rising (during the first few hours of light, early in the morning) for outdoor plants or just after the lights come on for indoor gardens. These periods are when the plants' absorption rates are highest, and they will have enough time to absorb the nutrients before the light gets too intense and hot. If you spray your plants with water in the middle of the day, you risk the water droplets acting like small magnifying glasses and burning your plants. On especially hot days, the leaves may also close their stomata, preventing them from absorbing the nutrients in the spray.

Many different forms of nutrients, including compost teas, mild organic fertilizers, and seaweed and kelp extracts, can be delivered to your plants by foliar feeding. You can create a foliar spray by mixing your preferred nutrients with water. It is important to use these items at a quarter or half the recommended dosage, erring on the side of using less rather than running the risk of your solution being too strong and potentially damaging your plants.

>>>> Lactic Acid Bacteria Serum

Lactic acid bacteria (LAB) help your plants to deal with stress, increase nutrient uptake, control pests and diseases, and can increase the quantity and quality of your yield. Once diluted, this serum can be used to water your plants and makes a great addition to compost and plant teas. It can also be used as a foliar spray or seed treatment to help combat fungal issues, such as damping off.

YIELD: ½ gallon (2 L)

What You Need

2 cups (470 ml) white rice

½ gallon (2 L) milk, any percentage

2 (1-gallon [3.8 L]) glass containers
(one container should have a wide mouth)

1. Wash and rinse your rice with water. Reserve the "rice wash," the starchy water that is left over after you've finished washing your rice. Pour the rice wash into the container without the wide mouth.

2. Cover the container with a piece of paper, towel, or cheesecloth and secure it around the container with a rubber band. Label it with the date.

3. Let the rice wash water sit for 3–5 days at room temperature, out of direct sunlight. You will know it is ready for the next step when there is a faint, sweet, fermented smell. If it smells sour, it has fermented too much, and you will have to start over.

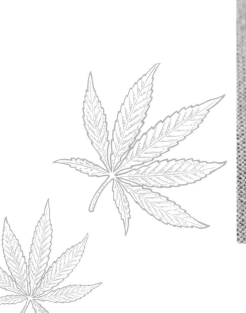

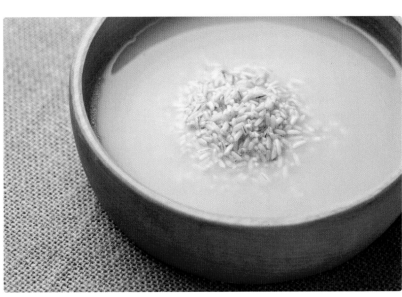

4. Pour the milk into a separate container. Add a generous ¾ cup (200 ml) of rice wash water to the milk. Cover the container with paper or a towel and secure it around the container with a rubber band. Label it with the date.

5. Leave the mixture for 48 hours at room temperature, out of direct sunlight. You will see the curds form and separate from the whey. The solid curds will float on the top of the mixture. There may be some sediment at the bottom of the container as well. The whey is the final product that you want and will be the liquid that makes up your serum. It will have a light beige or yellow color and may look slightly cloudy.

6. Cut the curds with a knife or a thin spatula. With a slotted spoon, gently pull out the curds and place them into the strainer or a separate bowl.

7. With a funnel and strainer, pour the mixture into a new container, leaving behind the sediment at the bottom.

8. Label the container and cover it with paper, a towel, or cheesecloth. Use a rubber band to secure the lid, and store it in the fridge. To use, refer to the table below to create a mixture that you can use for watering or as a foliar spray. The mixture will have a ratio of 1:1000 of LAB serum to water.

STORAGE: This can be kept in the fridge for approximately 6 months with the lid loosely capped. If you prefer to keep it at room temperature, add an equal amount of brown sugar (by weight), approximately 4 pounds (1.8 kg). The mixture should have a slightly sweet smell; if it starts to smell bad or rotten, discard it and make a new batch.

DILUTION RATIOS FOR LAB SERUM

Water Volume	Amount of LAB Serum to Add
½ gallon (2 L)	⅓ teaspoon (0.06 fl oz./2 ml)
1 gallon (3.8 L)	¾ teaspoon (0.13 fl oz./4 ml)
5 gallons (19 L)	1¼ tablespoons (0.64 fl oz./19 ml)
10 gallons (37.9 L)	2½ tablespoons (1.28 fl oz./38 ml)
25 gallons (95.6 L)	A scant ½ cup (3.2 fl oz./118 ml)

SOIL AMENDMENTS

A soil amendment is any material that is added to your soil to improve it. It can help increase the amount of organic matter in the soil and enhance its water retention, aeration, drainage, structure, and fertility. Many amendments act as fertilizers and stimulate microorganisms to break down organic matter and make the nutrients contained within it available for your plants. Most of the soil amendments described in this chapter are considered "slow-release fertilizers" because the organisms in the soil take a longer time to convert them to nutrients. For example, manure and compost can continue to release nitrogen into the soil for four years, sometimes more.

Many of the soil amendments listed on pages 73–80 are considered organic because they are composed solely of materials from living organisms, such as plants, animals, or algae, such as kelp. Under another definition, a soil amendment is also considered organic if it is produced with natural materials without any synthetic ingredients or chemicals.

Before You Buy

When purchasing amendments, it is important to ask yourself about the origin of these soil inputs and determine whether a product is something that you want to support and use. Consider if there is a way to procure the same benefits from another source or, even better, a product that you can grow, process, or make yourself. Look for resources that are close to you, readily available, and sourced from your own land or bioregion whenever possible, especially before you head to the store.

For plant-based products, like alfalfa pellets, check if the plants used to make these items were

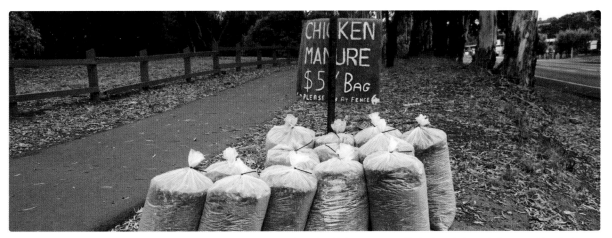

It is worth seeking out farmers in your area that sell soil amendments, such as the chicken manure on display here. Doing so helps support local businesses and makes it easier for you to ask questions about the sourcing and production of the amendments.

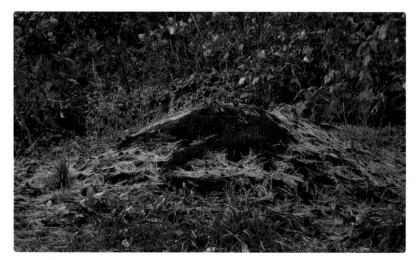
You don't always need to run to the store for soil amendments. For example, you can create compost in your backyard by using food scraps and other organic material that you might otherwise throw away.

grown organically, free from herbicides and pesticides. For some soil amendments, such as with bone and blood meal, manure, or even compost, consider the animals involved in the creation of these products and how they were treated. Even though the soil amendments themselves may be considered organic, the animals from which they were derived may not have been raised organically. For example, blood meal and feather meal often come from slaughterhouse animals subjected to factory farms and industrial agricultural practices. They may have been fed growth hormones, antibiotics, and various medications, and these substances may be in the final product that you are purchasing.

You should always ask the people or suppliers who are selling or making these products questions about sourcing. A reputable seller or supplier should be able to give you good answers. If they are hesitant to answer your questions or will not give answers at all, you may not want to use their products or resources.

You can search the internet for a list of products and amendments that are approved for organic agriculture. There are also several organizations that will certify various products as organic and approve them for organic agriculture, such as the Organic Materials Review Institute (OMRI), the United States Department of Agriculture (USDA), or the Canada Organic Regime (COR). Always do your own research on products and inputs that you are purchasing or bringing into your garden. It is important to make choices that feel right to you and are in line with your beliefs and ethics.

How to Use Soil Amendments

Once you have acquired various amendments, you will need to either add them to your soil or use them to make a potting mix. For indoor plants, you will simply incorporate the amendments by mixing them into a premade mix or use them when making a homemade mix.

In an outdoor garden, there are various ways to add amendments directly to your soil. One way is to simply apply them to the top of your soil and gently mix them into the top inch or two (2.5 or 5 cm) of soil, using your hands or a rake. This is known as top-dressing. Top-dressing works well for things such as compost, manure, alfalfa pellets, kelp meal, worm castings, wood chips, and mulch. Another method is to dig a large hole for your plant and place your amendments in layers inside the hole before planting. This works quite well for the first time that you plant cannabis plants in your garden. In subsequent years, you can place new plants using the same holes and top-dress your soil with amendments rather than disrupting the soil by digging a deep hole or tilling. Another option would be to add your amendments to the entire garden and then either turn them in with a garden fork or lightly till them in. With all these methods, it is best to put your amendments into the soil before you plant your cannabis and then, if needed, you can top-dress the soil once or twice over the course of the season.

Recommended Soil Amendments

I've described many different options for soil amendments here so that you can get a sense of different ones that are available and learn about their benefits. However, you do not need anywhere close to all these amendments to grow cannabis. We all have different resources available to us, depending on where we live, and we may not have access to or the money to purchase any of these products.

Alfalfa meal: Alfalfa is a great source of nitrogen and breaks down fast. You can use the fresh plant material or dried pellets. (If using pellets, make sure they are made with 100 percent alfalfa without any binding agents.) Alfalfa has a lot of potassium and trace minerals. It is best to top-dress with it or use it to make a plant tea (see page 132).

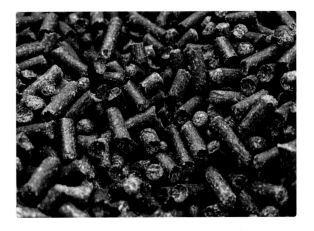

Bark mulch: Bark mulch works well for retaining moisture and supporting the fungal life in your soil. Almost any bark will do, but it is best to avoid black walnut as it contains a compound called juglone that can be toxic to some plants.

Biochar: Biochar, a type of charcoal that is used as a soil amendment, is an amazing substance that provides a home for microbes to live and thrive. It holds a variety of nutrients and retains water, enhancing long-term fertility and soil life. You can inoculate your biochar with microbes by brewing a compost or worm-casting aerated tea (see page 135) and then soaking the biochar in it. There are many ways to make biochar at home, or you can purchase it from a commercial manufacturer.

Blood meal: Blood meal is a powder made from dried animal blood, a by-product of the meat industry. It usually comes from cows and hogs. It is very high in nitrogen and iron, and contains many trace minerals. Be careful not to add too much—even ½ tablespoon (7.5 ml) for a 1-gallon (3.8-L) pot can be too much—and let it sit in the soil for a couple of weeks minimum before planting your plants. Mix it into the soil so it does not attract animals.

Bone meal: Bone meal is a slow-release source of phosphorus and nitrogen. It also adds calcium to your soil and can raise your soil's pH. Bone meal is a mixture of finely and coarsely ground bones and may contain other slaughterhouse by-products. It is often mixed with other high-nitrogen soil amendments, such as blood meal and manure, to create a well-balanced organic fertilizer.

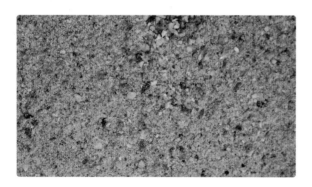

Coco coir: Coco coir can be a good additive to mix into soil mixes that will be used in pots. It does a good job of holding water and prevents the pH of the soil from becoming too low. As it breaks down, it also releases potassium, which is great for flowering cannabis. It is made from the hull of coconuts and, unlike other amendments such as peat moss, it does not have to be stripped from the land. In this sense, it may seem more environmentally friendly than peat moss. But because coco coir naturally has high-sodium content, it must be flushed or rinsed before it can be used. This requires a huge amount of fresh water, and the resulting runoff is not good for local environments. It also has to be shipped a long distance to reach North America (often from India or Sri Lanka), a process that burns a lot of fossil fuels.

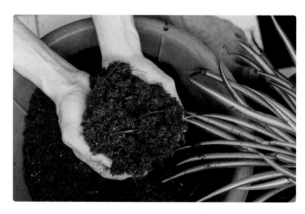

Compost: Compost is important for a number of reasons: It adds a type of organic matter called humus to your soil, contains nutrients for your plants to use, and is high in microbial life. It is an ideal slow-release fertilizer, and many growers will spread a thin layer (about 1 inch [2.5 cm] or so) over their garden beds each year. The macro- and micronutrient levels of your compost will vary depending on its ingredients. Many growers will also order large loads of compost to add nutrients and increase the fertility of their soil. The best way to obtain compost is to make it yourself and set up various compost bins and areas on your property. If you do not have the space to compost yourself, it is a good idea to search out high-quality compost that is available at your local garden center, greenhouse supply store, or specialty composting company.

Dolomite lime: Made of calcium and magnesium, dolomite lime buffers the pH of your soil, keeping it from falling too low or climbing too high. When added to heavy clay soils, it can also help to improve the workability of the soil.

Earthworm castings: Worm castings, or vermicast, is another term for manure from earthworms. The fresher you can get these, the better. Consider setting up your own vermicomposting unit and starting with a pound of red wigglers. They will eat your kitchen scraps and in turn become a rich source of microbial life. Earthworm castings contain a lot of water-soluble nutrients and are a great organic fertilizer or soil conditioner.

Farm animal manure: Animal manures are a rich source of nitrogen and mineral salts. Although various animal manures will differ slightly in their makeup and nutrient availability, one animal's manure is not necessarily better than another's. The best manure comes from your own animals; the second best manure is the type that is the closest to where you live and is free for the taking (and spreading!). Make sure they are well composted before using.

Feather meal: Feather meal slowly releases nitrogen and calcium and lasts a lot longer than blood meal. For those of you who hunt or live on a farm, you can make a similar fertilizer using hair and fur or hoof and horn.

Fish meal: Derived mostly from fish bones, fish meal slowly releases phosphorus and calcium. Like blood meal, it is generally mixed into the soil so that it does not attract animals. Some growers will mix the fish and bone meal together.

Greensand: Greensand is sandstone marine sediment that consists of a mixture of clay minerals. It is full of minerals that are released slowly into your soil and high in potassium. It can help build the structure of your soil.

Gypsum: Gypsum is made up of calcium and sulfur and is especially good to use in compacted clay soils. It slowly releases calcium and sulfur and seems to attract and increase beneficial fungal growth as well.

Humic acid ore: Humic acid ore is a catalyst that helps to make micronutrients, phosphorus, and potassium more bioavailable to your plants. It also helps to boost microbial life in the soil.

Kelp meal: Kelp meal contains more than sixty minerals or elements, and is a rich source of vitamins and amino acids. It is also high in potassium, and contains beneficial enzymes. Kelp contains a biostimulant that helps to reduce stress resulting from conditions such as transplant shock.

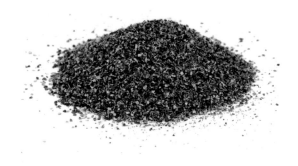

Oyster shell: Ground oyster shells are full of calcium and trace minerals that are released slowly and steadily throughout the growing season. These crushed shells also work well as an anchor for bacteria to adhere to and colonize.

Peat moss: Peat moss is a standard addition to many potting soils and is often used as the main ingredient (along with perlite) in many soilless mixes. It is soft, fluffy, and retains water well. It

has been the choice of growers for a long time and works quite well. Some people view peat as a renewable resource, but it is important to note that it has to be stripped from the northern parts of Canada at a great detriment to the natural ecosystem. It takes thousands of years to form extensive peat bogs, which consist of decomposed sphagnum moss and other plants, but only a few days to completely alter the local landscape through its extraction. These significant peat bog wetlands are home to all types of life, including plants, mammals, birds, and countless invertebrates. Although many in the peat industry would like you to believe this is not impacting these species, that is simply not the case. It is my hope that we can begin to limit and move away from using peat, and that larger growers will look for other options that are more environmentally friendly.

Rabbit manure: Rabbit manure is a great nitrogen-rich fertilizer. It is considered to be higher in nitrogen and other nutrients than most other common manures, though a rabbit produces less manure than a cow! It does not need to be composted for long (or at all) before being used. You can mix it into the soil or layer it on top. It helps with drainage and water retention, and improves soil structure.

Seabird and bat guanos: Seabird and bat guanos are made from the excrement of these animals. Some guano is higher in nitrogen, and others are high in phosphorus. Guano is also high in trace minerals. Note that it is often not harvested sustainably, as doing so can lead to the decline or destruction of bat and seabird colonies. It can also alter the shape of caves where bats live and cause bats to abandon them, leading to the loss of other species that rely on the bats. Consider using chicken manure instead, especially from free-range chickens that have been eating lots of insects.

Soft rock phosphate: This powder offers a slow-release source of phosphorus and sulfur and also helps to stabilize nitrogen in the soil so it does not off-gas into the air as ammonia.

Straw or hay mulch: A common form of mulch, hay and straw help retain moisture in your soil. They help break down additional organic matter, provide a habitat for fungi and microbes, and protect the soil from the sun, wind, and other elements.

Topsoil: Topsoil is just that—the top layer of soil. It should be a dark black color and is often used when people want to add soil to a rocky or gravelly area. The quality can vary, depending on where you get it from, but it can be a good one-time addition to a garden that does not already have a lot of topsoil.

Triple mix: *Triple mix* is a fancy name that generally describes a mix of topsoil, compost, and manure. It makes a great addition to your soil mix or garden beds. It can be more expensive than other amendments because it contains a few different ingredients. It may be cheaper to buy the ingredients separately.

Volcanic mineral fertilizers: There are many soil amendment products that are made from volcanic minerals. For example, Spanish River Carbonatite is a product made from volcanic carbonatite rock found near Sudbury, Ontario. Azomite is another option and is mined from a deposit in Utah. Products such as these can be a great way to add these micronutrients to your soil.

Wood chips: Wood chips can be used as mulch or to build up organic matter in your soil. They provide a great habitat for fungal life and a rich source of carbon for your plants.

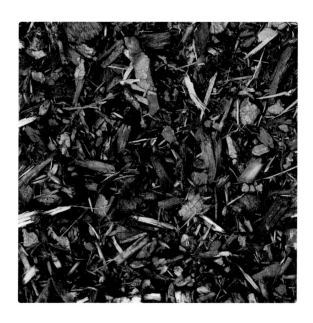

Mycorrhizal Products

Mycorrhizal fungi are underground wonders. They move through the soil with a threadlike structure and have an amazing symbiotic relationship with plants. When cannabis roots intertwine with mycorrhiza, the plant is more likely to reach its full potential and achieve vigorous growth and health. This symbiotic relationship between plants and these fungi has developed over millions of years of coevolution. Many researchers believe that neither fungi nor plants would have been able to successfully colonize the land without each other, and they have been working together ever since.

Only a few are known scientifically to be beneficial to cannabis. One of these types is known as arbuscular mycorrhiza fungi (AMF). These tiny fungi penetrate the plant's roots and create a branching structure called an arbuscle. It is in this structure that the fungi exchange nutrients, minerals, and water while receiving carbohydrates produced by the plant through photosynthesis. (How cool is that?) Because the mychorrhizae spread out through the soil and cover a larger surface area than the roots of the plant, they are able to secure and deliver nutrients to the plants from places that they would otherwise not come into contact with. When the plant needs more nutrients, it simply sends more carbohydrates down to its roots, which are delivered to the fungi in exchange for the nutrients. Mycorrhizal fungi are also able to free up phosphorus from the soil by secreting an enzyme that makes the phosphorus more bioavailable to the plant.

Healthy fungal life in your soil offers many additional benefits, including increased drought tolerance; a supply of nutrients that can be released when needed or stored for times of need; resistance against soil-borne pathogens, such as pythium, fusarium, and parasitic nematodes; and increased stress tolerance.

The earlier you can introduce mycorrhizal fungi to your plants' roots, the better. One way to introduce these fungi is to gather them from your landscape and use them to inoculate your garden beds. Look for areas (or wood chip piles) where there are small, white, threadlike mychorrhizae just under the soil surface. Gather some of this material and soil in a bucket, spread it in your garden, and cover with mulch.

There are also some myco products on the market that you can use to introduce these fungi to your garden. Many of these products come in a dehydrated powder. You add the powder directly to your pots or the ground when transplanting young cannabis plants. Make sure that your plants' roots will come into direct contact with the powder by sprinkling it into the pot or hole just before you finish transplanting them.

Once you've inoculated your plants, it is important to provide the right habitat for these fungi to thrive in your garden beds. Straw or hay mulch, wood chips, and sufficient moisture all help support fungi.

Amendments for Aeration

When growing cannabis in pots, it is important to have some kind of aeration in your soil mix. There are some additives you can use to help with this. Although perlite and vermiculite are not the best to use from a regenerative standpoint, they do serve this very useful purpose, especially if your plants will be spending a long time in pots.

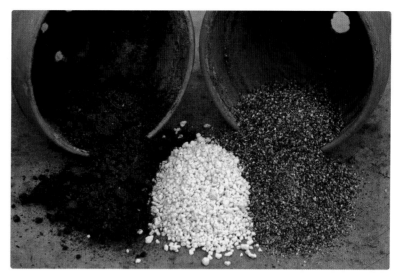

Examples of soil amendments that aerate soil. *From left to right:* peat, perlite, and vermiculate.

Perlite: Perlite is a volcanic glass 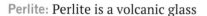 that has been heated at very high temperature. It is a nonrenewable resource and needs to be mined and processed to achieve the hard, expanded, and porous structure that makes it a useful addition to soil mixes. It does a great job of aerating soil, as well as providing a habitat for fungi and bacteria to colonize. Perlite is very light, has a neutral pH, and does not absorb water (though it will hold water along its surface). You can add it into your soil mix so that it comprises 10–15 percent of your mixture. Be careful not to breathe in perlite dust. It is best to wear a mask and gloves when working with this product.

Vermiculite: Vermiculite is another nonrenewable resource and is made by heating mica in large furnaces. It increases the aeration of soil (less so than perlite) and helps to hold water and nutrients (more so than perlite). It can expand and hold a lot of water and also provides a good place for fungi and bacteria to colonize. You can mix it into your soil mix at a 10 percent ratio. Some people will mix half perlite and half vermiculite for a combined 10–15 percent of their soil mix.

When growing cannabis outdoors in the ground, amendments to improve aeration are not as important. Most outdoor soils will aerate themselves just fine through earthworms, insects, and all the active microbial life.

If you have a heavy clay soil, it can be helpful to add some organic matter to improve aeration. Although many people recommend adding sand to heavy clay soils, this is not a good idea because, in most cases, it can mix with the clay and give your soil a cementlike consistency, the opposite of what you want. Instead, I recommend adding bark, sawdust, manure, leaf mold, compost, and peat moss to improve clay soil. Gypsum can also be used, especially if your soil is lacking or low in calcium. You can integrate this organic matter and gypsum directly into the soil by hand or by tilling. Clay soil will get harder with each round of tilling, so try to limit or eliminate the tilling after you have added your organic matter and be sure never to till it when it is wet. You may want to aerate the soil with a broad fork, which is less invasive than other tilling tools.

> **TIP:** If aeration is a problem for you, try not to walk on your beds to avoid compacting your soil, and always cover your soil with a thick layer of mulch.

BOTTLED NUTRIENTS

In the context of growing cannabis, bottled nutrients refer to any liquid fertilizer product that is sold in a store or a garden center. These products are mixed with water, and the mixture is poured into the soil. Many companies producing bottled nutrients formed during prohibition and marketed their products exclusively to cannabis growers. There are many bottled nutrients to choose from, especially if you go into any grow store in North America, and they will have fancy names and even fancier labels.

Do bottled nutrients work? Yes. Are they worth it? In most cases, no. In many ways, you are paying for the water in which the actual nutrients are suspended. I do, however, understand that many people may not have access to the space needed to nurture living soil or use the amendments outlined earlier. In these cases, it can be helpful to have some bottled nutrients on hand. If you are going to purchase these products, here are some things to consider:

- **When at all possible, choose organic.** Organic products are made using many of the additives and amendments listed on pages 73–80. Synthetic products are made using chemicals and salts.

- **Find out who owns the companies you are buying from.** Be aware that large corporations have been buying up many companies producing organic nutrients and other cannabis-related products. I believe it is best to support family-run and local businesses as much as possible.

- **Find out what is in the product, where it comes from, and why you will be using it.** Knowing what is in the product and where it comes from will allow you to make an ethical decision about whether this is a product and company that you want to support. It is also important to know why you will be using it, what nutrients it delivers to your plants, and if it is essential to your plants' nutritional needs.

- **Check if the product is specially formulated for a specific growing stage.** Cannabis nutrients and fertilizers are often formulated for vegetative growth and flowering. *Grow* will appear on labels for vegetative growth products, and *bloom* will appear on labels for products used for flowering.

- **Know that you can use a whole host of other micronutrient and supplements that you can find at your local grow store.** Some work well, and some not so much. They are not always necessary. You may find that you are already getting nutrients in other products or inputs that you have acquired or created yourself.

SOIL MIXES

Whenever possible, I recommend that you formulate and mix your own soil. This way, you will know exactly what is in it and why. If you can't do this, you can always research and purchase some premade soil mixes from a reputable company. When mixing your own soil, you have a number of options.

You can choose to make one type of soil or use different mixes for each stage of growth. For outdoor plants, you can add the ingredients for the soil mix directly into the holes that you will use to plant your cannabis. If you prefer not to mix your own soil, you can always purchase premixed "super soils."

Seed-Starting Mix

You want a seed-starting mix to be light and full of organic matter. The mix should make a small amount of nutrients available to the plants, stay moist and lofty, and avoid turning hard and dense when it dries out. You want the soil mix to allow your seeds to easily germinate and penetrate the soil surface without using too much energy. This will greatly improve the germination rate of your seeds.

Some mediums that work well for germination include premade peat moss mixes, screened

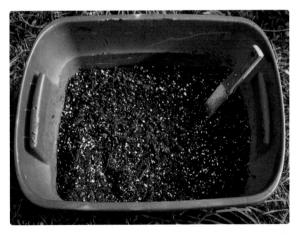

You always have the option to create any soil mix in advance and store it for later use in a bin or tarp, whether you plan to plant your cannabis in the ground or use the soil mix in containers.

compost mixed with coco coir or peat moss (especially if the compost is well decomposed and lofty), or a peat moss mixed with vermiculite and/or perlite. You can make and mix these mediums on your own. You will want the perlite or vermiculite (or a mixture of both) to equal approximately 10–15 percent of the final volume of your overall mix.

You can always use native soil instead of a seed-starting mix, as long as it is not too dense or rich in clay. These characteristics can make it hard for the seeds to break through the soil's surface. Consider adding some lofty organic matter, such as peat most or coco coir, to help make your native soil less dense. The key is for your final mix to be lightweight and lofty.

Soil Mixes for Outdoor Planting

You have a few soil mix options for outdoor plants. For each mix, you will need to dig a hole that is approximately 2½–3 feet (76–91 cm) deep and about 2–2½ feet (61–76 cm) in diameter. (If the hole needs to be a little smaller, that is fine.) You will dig one hole for each cannabis plant.

If you use the basic mix, your plant will benefit from extra nutrients from soil amendments over the course of the growing season. If you use the variation of the basic mix on page 83, additional nutrients are optional.

The advanced soil mix is best suited to a more advanced or motivated home grower, but if you use this mix, all you will have to do is water your plants as needed throughout the season. It is best if you can mix up each hole, and let it sit for at least a week or more before planting. You can give these plants some plant or compost teas over the growing season if you wish, but they should have everything they need from the amendments you've added in the hole. With some kind words and love, watch it grow!

In future growing seasons, you can plant your cannabis in the same holes or beds. It is up to you if you want to dig large holes again, or if you want to dig a hole just big enough to place your plant into it. Many of the amendments, such as volcanic minerals, soft rock phosphate, greensand, oyster shell, humic acid ore, and biochar, will stay in the soil and continue to feed your plants for a few years. If you want to add amendments to the soil, either you can use them to top-dress the soil around your plant and gently rake them into the soil surface, or you can dig into the soil and place them in a little deeper. You may also choose to add fewer amendments and mostly use compost and manure, and then cover the entire area with a nice layer of mulch. As you continue to build a healthy bed of living soil, you will not need to add many of these amendments to your soil as long as you are continuing to add organic matter, compost, and manure and mulching your beds. This is the ultimate goal with long-term regenerative cannabis growing.

>>>> Basic Soil Mix

What You Need

Shovel

Compost, manure, or a mixture of both

Triple mix or worm castings (optional)

Approximately 5 gallons (19 L) water

Mulch of your choice

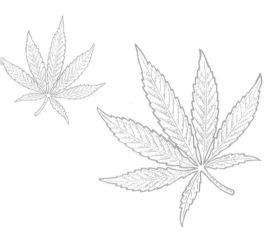

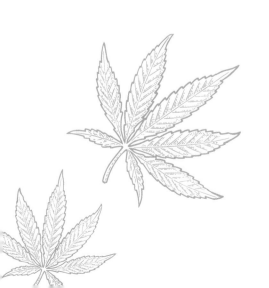

1. Add approximately 3 shovelfuls each of native soil and compost or manure to the bottom of the hole and stir until well mixed. If you like, you can add one shovelful of triple mix or worm castings or a shovelful of each into this soil mix as well.

2. Keep adding equal parts of native soil and compost or manure, and mixing until you fill the hole. If you have extra soil, you can make a berm around the outside edge of the hole. This creates a well that will aid in the absorption of water.

3. Dig a small hole just big enough for your plant, and place your plant in this hole.

4. Slowly pour the water on the top of the hole around the plant so that it seeps into the ground and does not run off the soil surface away from the hole.

5. Cover the entire top of the hole with hay, straw, wood chips, or another mulch of your choice.

....

VARIATION

What You Need

Shovel

Compost, manure, or a mixture of both

Triple mix or worm castings (optional)

1 cup (240 ml) soil amendment with phosphorus, such as bone meal, fish meal, or bat or seabird guano

1 cup (240 ml) soil amendment with nitrogen, such as blood meal, feather meal, or alfalfa meal

2 cups (470 ml) volcanic minerals (such as Spanish River Carbonatite or Azomite)

Approximately 5 gallons (19 L) water

Mulch of your choice

1. Add approximately 3 shovelfuls each of native soil and compost or manure to the bottom of the hole and stir until well mixed. If you like, you can add one shovelful each of triple mix or worm castings into this soil mix as well.

2. Add the soil amendment with phosphorus and approximately 2 shovelfuls each of native soil and compost or manure.

3. Repeat step 2 but add the soil amendment with nitrogen. Stir until well mixed.

4. Repeat step 2 again but add the soil amendment with volcanic minerals. Stir until well mixed.

5. Continue filling the hole with a mixture of native soil, compost, and/or manure until you fill the hole. If you have extra soil, you can make a berm around the outside edge of the hole. This creates a well that will aid in the absorption of water.

6. Dig a small hole just big enough for your plant and place your plant in this hole.

7. Slowly pour the water on the top of the hole around the plant so that it seeps into the ground and does not run off the soil surface away from the hole.

8. Cover the entire top of the hole with hay, straw, wood chips, or another mulch of your choice.

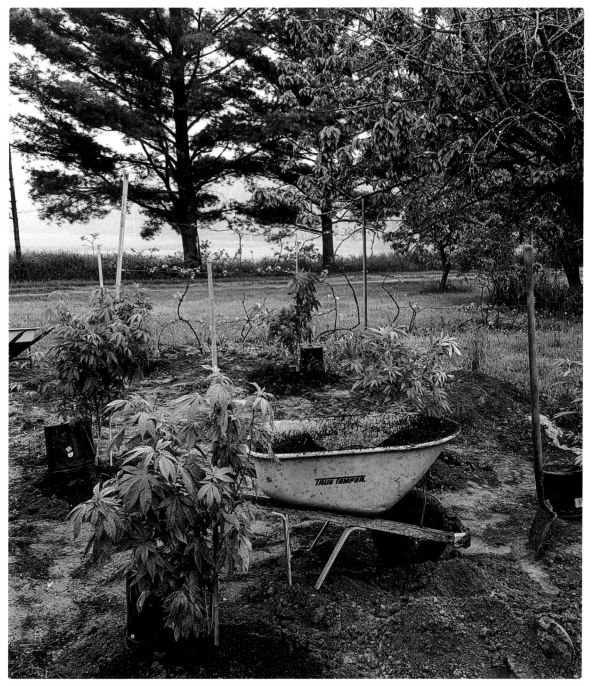

Adding and layering the ingredients of each soil mix into the holes where you will plant your cannabis will give your plant's roots direct access to the nutrients in the mix.

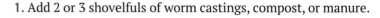

>>>>> Advanced Soil Mix

What You Need

Shovel

Worm castings, compost, manure, or a mixture of all three

1 cup (240 ml) blood meal

1 cup (240 ml) bone meal

2 cups (470 ml) volcanic minerals (such as Spanish River Carbonatite or Azomite)

2 cups (470 ml) biochar

1 cup (240 ml) humic acid ore (powder or granulated)

1 cup (240 ml) feather meal

1 cup (240 ml) fish meal

1 cup (240 ml) kelp meal

1 cup (240 ml) oyster shell

2 cups (470 ml) greensand

1 cup (240 ml) rock phosphate

1–2 tablespoons mycorrhiza powder

Approximately 5 gallons (19 L) water

2 cups (470 ml) alfalfa pellets

Mulch of your choice

Note: You can use any soil amendment that provides a good source of nitrogen source instead of the blood and bone meal.

1. Add 2 or 3 shovelfuls of worm castings, compost, or manure.

2. Add the blood meal and bone meal, along with the volcanic minerals, biochar, and humic acid ore.

3. Add in 3 shovelfuls of your native soil. Mix until evenly distributed.

4. Repeat steps 1 and 3. Add the feather meal, fish meal, kelp meal, oyster shell, greensand, and rock phosphate.

5. Add 3 or 4 shovelfuls of your native soil, and mix this layer thoroughly with the contents of the hole.

6. Repeat steps 1 and 5. Mix the layer of native soil thoroughly.

7. Continue to fill the hole using a mixture of 2 parts native soil to 1 part worm castings, compost, or manure. If you have extra soil, you can make a berm around the outside edge of the hole. This creates a well that will aid in the absorption of water. If possible, let the hole sit for at least one week before planting.

8. When you are ready to plant your cannabis plant, dig a new hole that is a little bigger than the pot with your plant.

9. Sprinkle the mycorrhiza powder into the hole and then put your plant into the hole. Cover the hole gently but firmly with soil.

10. Slowly pour the water on the top of the hole around the plant so that it seeps into the ground and does not run off the soil surface away from the hole.

11. Sprinkle the alfalfa pellets on the soil surface a few inches from the stem of your plant. Cover this area with mulch.

12. Cover the entire top of the hole with hay, straw, wood chips, or another mulch of your choice.

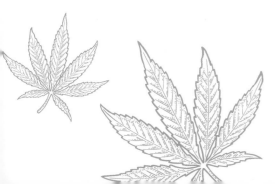

Soil Mix for Container Plants

YIELD: 18 gallons (68.1 L)

When mixing soil recipes for container plants, you can use a large tote or tarp to contain all the listed ingredients and then mix them together. You can scale this recipe up or down to produce a larger or smaller amount of soil, depending on how much you need. Once you have procured all the ingredients, simply follow the mixing instructions on the next page and you will be well on your way to making your own high-quality, organic growing medium.

If you are growing cannabis in pots or containers (and outdoor beds), it is important to recycle your soil and continue to build it up by adding new amendments as you continue to garden. Many indoor growers will reuse their soil dozens of times and often remark that it gets better with age. You may choose to plant right back in the same pots (or beds) and add some amendments to the top layer of soil. (This is my first choice.) Another option is to dump the soil from your pots into a large container and mix up a whole new batch of soil. If you do not plan to grow more plants indoors, you can add your used soil to existing garden beds outside or sprinkle it over your lawn so that it can go back into the earth.

Base Mix

8 gallons (30.2 L) high-quality organic soil mix (see recipe on page 88 to make your own)

2 gallons (7.6 L) coco coir fiber, rinsed thoroughly with cold water, or 2 gallons (7.8 L) premade soil mix if rinsed coir is unavailable

4 gallons (15 L) perlite (with small nuggets) or 50/50 mix of vermiculite and perlite

4 gallons (15 L) earthworm castings, compost, or a mixture of both

Soil Amendments

½ cup (118 ml) greensand

½ cup (118 ml) ground oyster shells (or 1½ cups if crushed)

1 cup (240 ml) powdered dolomite lime

½ cup (118 ml) blood meal

2 cups (470 ml) feather meal

2 cups (470 ml) bone meal

¼ cup (60 ml) powdered soft rock phosphate (¾ cup rock phosphate granular, if powdered is not available)

½ cup (118 ml) powdered gypsum (or 1 cup [240 ml] if granular)

3 cups (710 ml) kelp meal

4 cups (946 ml) alfalfa meal

½ cup (118 ml) volcanic minerals, such as Spanish River Carbonatite or Azomite

¼ cup (60 ml) granular humic acid ore, such as Black Earth Humic

4–6 cups (946 ml–1,400 ml) manure

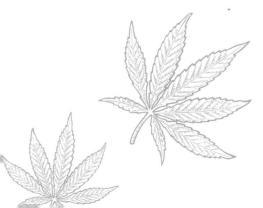

1. Add the base mix to your large tote, bin, or tarp. Add the soil amendments on top of the base mix.

2. Stir and mix thoroughly with a shovel or your hands.

3. Sprinkle this mix with approximately 5 gallons (19 L) of water or until saturated.

4. Let this mix sit and "cook" for 2–4 weeks in a dry place before using it for planting.

STORAGE: Store extra soil in a barrel or tote with a lid so that it does not get rained or snowed on. It can be stored inside or outside.

HOMEMADE ORGANIC SOIL MIX

YIELD: 8 gallons (30.2 L)

4 gallons (15 L) topsoil

2 gallons (7.6 L) native soil from your garden or, if this is not available, topsoil or triple mix

2 gallons (7.6 L) coco coir fiber, rinsed thoroughly with cold water, or peat moss

1. Add the ingredients into a large tote, bin, or tarp.

2. Stir and mix thoroughly with a shovel or your hands.

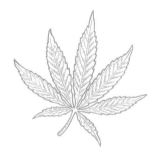

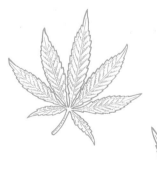

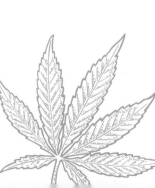

FAQS & TROUBLESHOOTING

Q: Do I need to purchase all these amendments?

A: No, not at all. The lists on pages 73–80 are intended to give you an idea of the various options as well as what they are used for. You can try any combination of amendments, depending on what you have available and what you can purchase or make on your own. Pick what works for you. You can always try new amendments and recipe variations in future years.

Q: Can I just plant my cannabis directly in my native soil?

A: Go for it. Your plants will most likely do better with some extra amendments added, but they may do just fine in your soil, too. There is no harm in trying. If you notice any nutrient deficiencies, you should be prepared to add the required amendments that will bring your plants back into health. Look through the list of amendments and see what is available to you in your local area. It is always best to either add what you can before you plant or be prepared to treat a nutrient deficiency, especially a deficiency in nitrogen, since cannabis uses a lot of it in the vegetative stage.

You can just use native soil for indoor plants, too, but I would recommend adding something such as perlite or vermiculite to aerate your soil, plus some soil amendments. Soil varies tremendously, depending on where you live. There is nothing wrong with trying to grow some plants in pots in your native soil, but carefully observe your plants for any problems. If it works out, that's great. If not, take note of what you can do differently with your soil the following year.

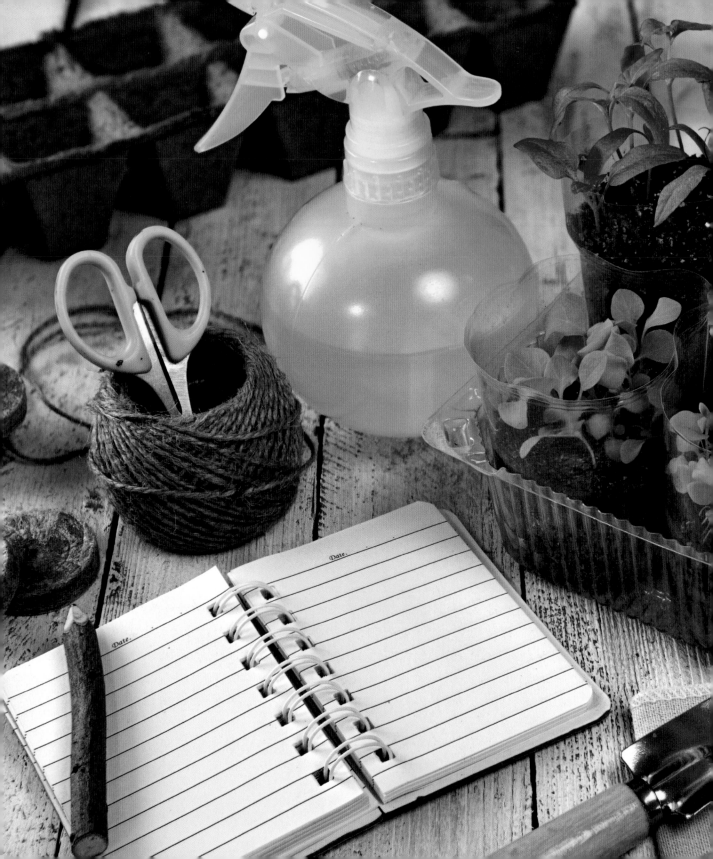

Date.

Date.

CHAPTER 6

< Essential Plant Care Techniques >

When growing cannabis, it is important to provide your plants with everything they need to be strong, healthy, and disease- and pest-resistant. In this chapter, we will talk about how to design an effective scouting and observation regimen in your garden (see below), when to transplant your plants to keep them from getting root-bound (see page 98), how to water them effectively (see page 96), and more. Even if you think you have a black thumb, I hope to impart valuable tools and skills that can turn that thumb green. Be patient and methodical while working with your plants, and soon you will acquire the necessary skills.

OBSERVE YOUR PLANTS

There is a saying that summarizes the best approach to plant care: "The best fertilizer for a crop is the shadow of the farmer. The more frequently it is applied, the better the likely outcome." This age-old axiom rings true not only for vegetables, herbs, and agricultural crops, but also for cannabis. If we are not observing and watching our plants constantly, we may miss the subtle clues, signs, and messages that they broadcast about their health, wellness, and vitality. The more time you spend with your plants and the more you get to know each one as a unique

individual, the more quickly you will be able to notice when they need your help and provide what they need to remain healthy and vibrant.

Although many of us would like to spend our entire day in the garden tending to our plants, this is simply not possible for most. I suggest that you schedule time to interact with your plants every day. Make a habit to stroll through the garden each morning with your tea or coffee. Take a break in the middle of the day and visit your plants. As soon as you get home from work, grab your favorite beverage and check out your plants. You may be surprised by how you both react to this experience. Many gardeners find this time

LEFT One of the most important habits to develop for a home grower is writing in a plant journal. Your observations will create an invaluable resource that can help you detect problems early and guide you in future growing seasons.

< 91 >

to be very meditative. Your visits to the garden can be a time to relax, forget your busy schedule, and tune into the natural world. Plants are great at teaching you how to slow down, relax, and be present in the moment. Enjoy this time, and be grateful for the space that it provides.

Here are a few things that you can do while you walk and move through your garden:

- Look for signs of health and disease in your plants. Observe them closely and note any changes that are happening from day to day. Record your observations in a notebook (see "Keep a Plant Journal," page 93).

- Look for pests and beneficial insects that may be living on or moving around on your cannabis plants.

- Learn to identify and understand the biology and behavior of the insects, mammals, birds, reptiles, and amphibians in your garden and throughout your bioregion. Get some field guides or books from your local library, or do some research online to get to know the habits, biology, and behaviors of these various species with which you share space.

- Get to know the other plants, trees, and shrubs that are growing in your garden, on your land, and in your neighborhood.

Are they edible or medicinal? Do they have practical uses, and what role do they play in the ecosystem?

- Find out where your water comes from and where it goes.

- Pay attention to the weather, the clouds, and how conditions change throughout the day, week, month, and season. How do these changes affect your plants?

- Meditate and connect with not only your plants but also the land itself. Ask yourself the sacred question: What happened or is happening here and what can I learn from it? You'll begin to see and, more importantly, feel how you are interconnected to all things in nature.

- Sit quietly and observe the life that comes and goes from your cannabis plants. Use all your senses to experience your garden. Get out of your head, and live in the moment. I like to say, "Lose your mind and come to your senses."

- Find out who the indigenous people in your area are. They have lived in this area for thousands of years and are the original stewards and caretakers of that land. Learn how they looked after the land and took care of it for future generations.

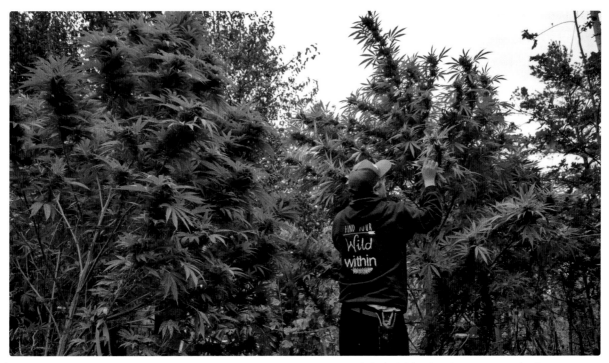

Cannabis thrives best when its caretakers keep a close eye on it. Inspecting your plants each day and giving them the proper care and maintenance through the growing season will pay off come harvest time. Here I am seeing whether this plant is ready for harvesting.

By following some or all of the practices listed above (and creating more on your own), you will begin to understand your space and your role within it on a deeper level. Nature is always teaching—that is part of the beauty of working with natural systems. We can always learn more about the complex relationships that connect all life on earth.

Keep a Plant Journal

It is a good idea to get a notebook and start a plant journal. A plant journal is a place where you can record your observations about your garden and dates of major events, transitions, and happenings in the life of your plants. If you prefer, you can keep a journal on your phone. I cannot tell you how beneficial this process will become for future growing seasons. No matter how hard you try, you will not remember everything that happens in your garden. By recording your observations, you will create a living record of your garden, to which you can refer year after year. You will begin to see patterns form and develop a better understanding of how cannabis grows in your environment and the proper timing for tasks such as transplanting and harvesting. You can observe how certain cultivars perform compared to others, track weather patterns, and note how you handled challenges for future reference.

I recommend that you write in this journal as much as you can, even if it's just a few bullet points each day. If possible, write a longer entry once a week. Here is some information that you will want to record:

- The time and date when you plant your seeds, transplant seedlings into bigger pots, move your plants outside, and plant them in the ground

- The length of time it takes for your seeds to germinate

- Fertilizer and nutrient feeding schedules

- Soil preparations and the soil amendments that you are using

- How each cultivar performs, including their height and growth patterns

- The size of your plants at certain times of year

- The date when your plants begin to show signs of their sex

- If you're growing indoors, the type of lights you use and how your plants respond to them

- If you're growing outdoors, the weather patterns in your area, including the first and last frost dates, high and low temperatures, storms, wind direction, and amount of precipitation

- The beginning of the flowering for each cultivar

- Descriptions of any pests, diseases, and/or nutrient deficiencies and how you deal with them

- Descriptions of any beneficial insects and your observations of them

- The date and time of your harvest and which plants were finished first

- How long you dried and cured each plant

Keeping a journal may seem like a simple task that you do not need to do, but trust me. It is a great tool for any grower, and if you ask around, you will find that all the best growers have a routine for recording information about their plants.

WATERING

Water helps to transport nutrients from the roots of the plants to the stems, leaves, and flowers, and is needed for photosynthesis. After water is distributed to the stems, leaves, and flowers of the plant, some of it will leave the plant via the stomata in the leaves, along with waste products—a process called "transpiration." The remaining water carries starches and sugars manufactured by photosynthesis back down to the roots. Water is essential to the growth of your plants, and it is important to learn how to provide the right amount of it.

Evaluating Your Water

The water from one area may be a little different than water from another. Some water is "hard," meaning that it contains a lot of minerals, such as calcium and magnesium. The more total dissolved solids (TDS) that you have in your water, the harder it is. The unit of measurement for TDS is parts per million (ppm). To find out whether your water is hard or soft, you can call your local water authority, and they will be able to let you know what the conditions of your tap water are. You can also purchase a TDS meter.

Hard water is not much of an issue when growing plants in the ground or in living soil. Generally speaking, the microorganisms in the soil will act as a filter and help to buffer the pH of the water. If you grow indoors, hard water increases the risk of nutrient lockout—the inability of the roots to take up the nutrients that your plants need for optimum growth. The risk is particularly high if your water has a TDS measurement of 400–500 ppm and you are using bottled nutrients. If hard water is a problem for you, there are a few solutions. You can collect and use rainwater for watering or use distilled water. Some growers, especially those growing cannabis on a large scale, set up a reverse osmosis or carbon filtration system, which removes most of the total dissolved solids from the water, but this is neither economical nor necessary for

most home growers. You can also look for bottled nutrients that are designed specifically to be used with hard water.

If you live in a town or city in North America, your water is likely to be chlorinated. Although chlorine in small amounts is essential for photosynthesis (among other functions), the levels of chlorine in municipal water are often high enough to affect plant growth negatively. For this reason, it is best to fill up your pails or buckets with water and let them sit out for 24 to 48 hours before using it for watering to let the chlorine evaporate. If you are not going to use this water within a couple of days after the chlorine has evaporated, it is a good idea to cover the top of the bucket with a lid.

It is a good idea to check the pH of your water and runoff (the excess water that has passed

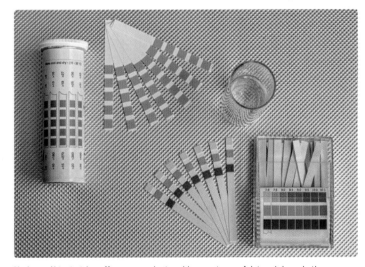

Various pH test strips offer a convenient and low-cost way of determining whether your water is alkaline or acidic. If you plan on testing your water regularly, I recommend investing in a digital pH meter.

through your soil) every now and then, especially when growing indoors and in pots while using bottled nutrients. If your water and soil pH are out of balance, you can run into many issues, including nutrient lockout. Levels of pH are measured on a scale from 0 to 14, with 7 being neutral. A reading between 0 and 7 indicates that your water is acidic, and a reading between 7 and 14 indicates that it is alkaline. You want your water to fall between 6.3 and 6.5 when using soil and soilless mixes. If your water does not fall within these parameters, you can adjust it by using special solutions (such as pH down and pH up) from your local grow store.

The temperature of your water is as important as the pH. Your water should be around room temperature, 65°F–80°F (18.5°F–27°C). Your plants do not like the water to be too hot or too cold. You can check the temperature of your water with a thermometer, or you can fill up a bucket or two with cold water and then leave it overnight to come to the proper temperature.

Best Watering Practices

It is best to let your plants almost dry out between waterings. They do not like to be dry or wet for too long, so try to maintain a balance between wet and dry cycles. Different size plants and pots will dry out at different times, so you may not need to water every plant in your garden at the same time.

Watering is done in a number of ways. You may choose to purchase a watering can from a local garden center or simply use a bucket with a small jar or pitcher to deliver water to your plants. In some cases with large plants in the ground, you may give them a large amount of water by pouring it directly out of a 5-gallon (19-L) bucket onto the soil. Using a hose is a great option that is less labor-intensive. You can purchase extended handles, called wands, that make watering in hard-to-reach places easier or nozzles that regulate the flow of water from your garden hose through various different spray patterns. Whatever tool you choose, be sure that the water permeates the soil at the base of your plant and does not run off and drain away from the root area.

For plants that are growing in the ground outdoors, be sure to pay attention to the amount of rainfall that you are getting, the air temperature, and the size of your plants. If you live in an arid, dry region that does not get a lot of rain, you will need to water your plants more often. A large, healthy, and fast-growing plant (4 feet [1.2 m] or more tall) can use a lot of water. It is a good idea to water your plants every 3–4 days if there is no rainfall between waterings. If it is hot and sunny outside, you will likely need to water every 2–3 days. Plants less than 4 feet tall will need less frequent watering. As always, pay attention to what your plants are telling you.

Each time you water your indoor plants, make sure that you fully saturate the soil in the pot. It is best to water until you see some water beginning to drip through the drainage holes in the bottom of the pot. This is one way that you can tell that the soil in the pot is approaching the saturation point.

With many soilless mediums, such as peat moss, the water will often flow directly through the substrate and run out of the drainage holes in the bottom of the pot. If this is the case, you can use a catchment tray and allow the pot to sit in the excess water. In half an hour or so, the medium will suck up some of that water into the dry soil. However, avoid letting your plant sit in this water for too long or the roots can drown and die back. You can add a little water at a time, giving it a better chance to fully soak into the soil without the risk of drowning the roots.

One of the most common mistakes new growers make is overwatering. Make sure you do not kill your plants with "water-kindness." Get used to letting them dry out a little between waterings, as they do not like a root system that is soggy all the time. As your plants grow, you will start to see a pattern for how much water they need and how quickly they dry out. When your plants are in the ground, pay attention to the weather conditions and make note of how long it has been between rainfalls to decide when to water.

The nice thing about growing outdoors and in the soil is that, more often then not, the water will drain away through the ground, and there is a much lower chance of overwatering. If you have heavy clay soils that do not drain very well, you will need to water less often and may want to look

at amending the soil in order to improve drainage (see page 71). Conversely, if you have very sandy soils that drain quickly, you may need to water your plants more often and may want to consider adding more organic matter into your soil that will help increase water retention.

If you are growing your plants in containers, I always tell people to pick up and feel the weight of your pots right after you water and when they have dried out and are ready for another watering. By getting to know what a wet pot and a dry pot feels like, you'll be able to tell when your plant needs water simply by lifting the pot, thereby avoiding overwatering. Do not just rely on what you see, as the top layer of soil might look dry but the bottom layers might still have moisture.

When a plant is in need of water, the lower leaves will begin to droop. As it continues drying out, the drooping will move up the plant. Eventually, the whole plant will begin to sag and drop down toward the ground. A sagging plant will come back to health with a drink or two, but you want to avoid this as much as possible. It causes undue stress on your plant and can also lead to dry pockets in your soil that do not become sufficiently saturated with subsequent watering.

TRANSPLANTING AND POTS

Most people will grow their cannabis in pots for a short time before transplanting them into the ground. Others will choose to grow their plants in pots for the entire growing season, perhaps because of a lack of garden space, nosy neighbors, or limited access to an outdoor area. Regardless of your reason for keeping your cannabis in a pot, it is very important to make sure that your plants have adequate space for a healthy root system to develop. Healthy roots will lead to healthy plants.

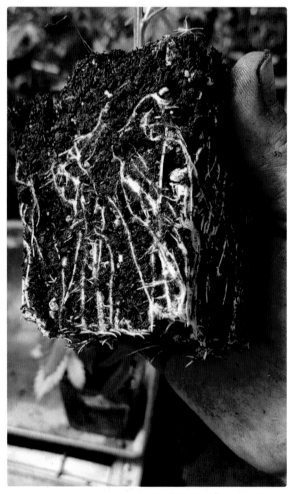

This cannabis plant has healthy white roots with no signs of being root-bound. It is ready to be transplanted into the ground or a larger pot.

Choosing the Correct Size Pot

If your plants are left for too long inside a small pot, they will become root-bound, which slows their growth. When a plant becomes root-bound, the roots become restricted by the size of the pot, wrapping around one another and the bottom of the pot. They will not be able to absorb nutrients nearly as well as they could in a larger pot that would give them more space. You will notice that your root-bound plant will have less branching and slow vertical growth. (Healthy plants will grow branches that extend beyond the sides of your pot.) Another sign that a plant is root-bound is that it dries out quickly and needs daily watering. If this is the case, you should transplant it as soon as possible. If left unattended, your root-bound plants may become sick and start to show signs of nutrient deficiencies.

While you do not want your pots to be too small, you also do not want them to be too big. If you transplant your plants into a pot that is too big when they are young, it will make it hard for your plants to use all the water in the soil. The plants could become oversaturated, resulting in stunted growth and yellowing leaves. I recommend using a 4-inch (10-cm) size pot for plants once they are transplanted from their cell packs. If you do not have cell packs, you can plant your seeds directly into the 4-inch (10-cm) pots. As your plants grow, the subsequent pots you transplant them into should be about two or three times larger than the pots they are leaving.

To make sure your final pot is the proper size, a general rule is to have a minimum size of 1 gallon (3.8 L) for every foot (30 cm) of vertical growth. For example, if you expect your plant to reach a height of 5 feet (1.5 m), you should plant it in a pot that is at least 5 gallons (19 L). For your final transplant, I recommend finding a pot that is a minimum of 5–10 gallons (19–37.9 L). Go with the largest size pot that you can accommodate in your space. (Just keep in mind that a larger pot may make it hard to physically move your plants around over the course of the growing season.) The more space your plant has to spread its roots, the larger your potential yield will be come harvest season. The larger pots will also help keep the soil moist for longer, allow it to dry out less quickly, and help you to spend less time watering. It's a good idea to spread a layer of mulch (made with straw, hay, or wood chips) on top of the soil.

When to Transplant

When you transplant your plants at the optimal time, you allow the roots to spread out through the soil in the new pot. If you time each transplant perfectly, your plants will not suffer transplant shock (or suffer very little from it), allowing them to continue growing with strength and vigor.

Before transplanting, make sure that your plants are healthy and growing vigorously, and have a strong root system. One way you can check on the health of your roots is to place your hand over the top of the pot and then tip it upside down. Gently squeeze the pot and tap the bottom to allow the soil to slip out of the pot. If the soil is loose and wants to fall apart, your plant is not ready to transplant. If the soil comes out easily in one intact piece and there are lots of roots at the bottom of the pot, then it is ready to be up-potted (transplanted into a bigger pot).

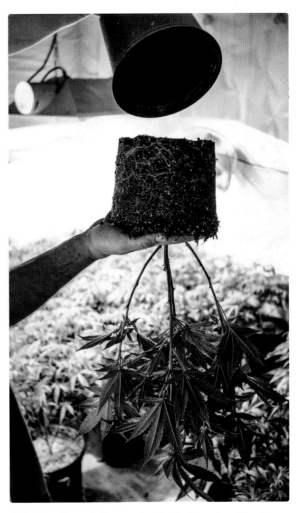

The best way to see whether your plant has healthy roots and is not becoming root-bound is to remove your plant from its container by turning it upside down.

I prefer to up-pot plants during the initial stages of growth from seedling to the early vegetative stage. It is best to avoid transplanting plants at all during the flowering stage. Because photosynthesis, nutrient uptake, and growth slow down after transplanting, you want to move your plants into their final home at least 1–2 weeks, preferably longer, before the flowering phase begins so that your plants have time to recover from the transplant. Otherwise, your plants will spend some of their energy sending out roots to fill up the new container and recovering from transplant shock, which will take away resources that would have been put into flower production and lower your yields.

TRANSPLANT SHOCK

Transplant shock is the stress that a plant experiences after it is moved from one pot to another or from a pot into the ground. All plants will experience some form of transplant shock, but these effects can be mitigated when transplanting is done properly and at the right time. Some signs of transplant shock in cannabis are slowed growth, yellowing or wilted leaves, branch or leaf die-off, reddening of the stem, flimsy growth, and an overall unhealthy appearance.

If your plants show any of these symptoms, they should recover in about a week or so. If this is not the case, you will need to investigate other potential causes for your plant's condition, such as a nutrient deficiency or excess, over- or underwatering, soil pH imbalances, and more. To avoid or limit transplant shock, make sure that your plants do not become root-bound and follow the transplanting tips on page 101.

Steps to Successful Transplanting

What You Need

Soil

Water

Pot for the transplanted plant

Trowel

1. Before starting, make sure that you have enough soil to fill your pot and an additional amount set aside. This additional amount should be a quarter of the amount that you're using for your pots. For example, if you are planning to transplant four plants, reserve 1 extra pot of soil. Moisten the additional soil with pH-balanced water. (This premoistened soil will be used in step 6.)

2. Fill the pot approximately halfway to the top with your chosen soil medium.

3. Water the soil in the new pot with pH-balanced water. Water the plant as well, if it is dry.

4. Remove the plant from its old pot by placing your hand flat across the top of the pot with the stem between two fingers. Gently squeeze the pot and tap the bottom so that the plant comes smoothly out of the pot.

5. Place this plant into the new pot so that it sits about 2 inches (5 cm) below the top of the pot. You may need to add or take out soil.

6. Fill in the space around the new plant with the premoistened soil (from step 1) and gently press it down lightly to avoid leaving any air pockets around the root ball.

7. Water the plant until a little water begins to come out of the bottom of the pot.

8. Place the freshly transplanted plants on the edge of your indoor garden (away from the full strength of your light source) or in a slightly shady spot outdoors for a couple of days until you notice fresh growth. Once you see fresh growth, you can put them back under the full intensity of your lights or the sun.

Transplanting Tips

- Water your plants one day before transplanting, and water them after transplanting.

- Transplant your plants in the afternoon or close to lights-out time. This gives them a little more time to recover from the process and will help to alleviate transplant shock.

- Use a well-balanced and well-draining soil, and avoid packing the soil too tightly. It is ideal to use a similar soil medium in the new pot for roots and water to penetrate the new medium as well as they did in the old medium.

- Be careful not to disturb or damage the roots, especially with young plants. If your plant is root-bound, gently massage and break apart the roots that have coiled around the bottom of the pot. This will allow them to spread out more easily into the new soil after transplanting.

- Know that transplanted plants require less nitrogen and potassium and a little more phosphorus for root development. They will also benefit from any form of vitamin B_1.

- Encourage new root growth. You may want to consider using a willow bark tea (see page 102) or a kelp or seaweed extract so your plant will settle into its new home quickly. To use kelp or seaweed extract, mix the extract with water using the instructions provided by the manufacturer.

>>>>> Willow Bark Tea

This tea acts as a natural root growth enhancer after transplanting. It can also be used to encourage roots to form on clones.

What You Need

Small willow tree branch (from any member of the genus *Salix*)*

Knife

Water

---

*Look for a local willow that grows in your area. Examples of some species you may find include *Salix bebbiana* (Bebb willow) or *Salix nigra* (black willow). You want roughly a handful of bark per cup (240 ml) of water.

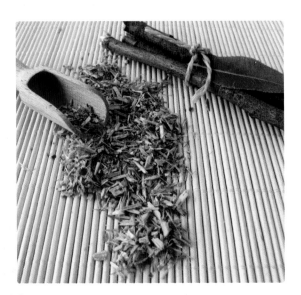

1. Harvest a small branch or a branch from a young sapling about as thick as your thumb and 18–24 inches (45–61 cm) long. Peel off the bark with the knife.

2. Bring a small pot of water to a boil and then take it off the heat. Add the willow bark to the hot water.

3. Cover the pot and let it sit overnight or for approximately 6–8 hours.

4. Strain the tea through a sieve or cheesecloth into a clean jar. Compost the willow bark.

5. To use the tea, create a diluted solution with a ratio of 1 part willow bark tea to 10 parts water. Use this to water your plants. You can add the diluted tea for the first two waterings after transplanting to encourage root growth. The willow bark tea can be stored in the fridge for approximately 1 week or can be frozen indefinitely. It's best to use fresh tea whenever possible.

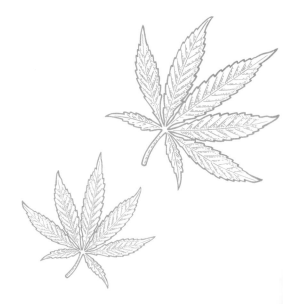

MAINTENANCE

Throughout the growing season, you will need to perform some additional tasks besides watering and transplanting to keep your plants healthy. The more time and care you give your plants, the more healthy they will be, and they will also be better equipped to fend off any potential issues, such as drought, pests, and disease. This extra work on plant maintenance is essential, and it will ultimately lead to bigger yields come harvest season.

Mulching

Mulch is any material that covers the soil between and around your plants. It keeps soil protected and covered; helps it retain moisture; protects the integrity of your soil from erosion, drought, and direct sunlight; and creates a beautiful environment for microbes and fungi to thrive. It will also break down and add organic matter to your soil, and as it decomposes you will have to keep adding it to the top of your soil. I highly recommend that you spread mulch on your garden, as it will build the integrity of your soil and help your plants grow bigger and stronger. Straw, hay, and wood chips are all good choices for mulch, and they can be used both indoors and out.

Plant Supports

As your plants grow taller, it will be important to support them in some way to help them remain upright, especially with all the dense, heavy flowers that will come with the flowering cycle. There are many options when it comes to supporting your plants: bamboo or wooden stakes, straight tree branches, metal T-bars, high-tensile wire, wire fence, cages, trellis netting, and more.

Some cultivars with thick stems and strong structures may not need much additional support, while others will benefit from having it. For a new grower, I recommend that you provide some support to all your plants. I have found that plants with adequate external support will grow bigger and produce heavier flowers.

No matter what method you choose for supporting your plants, it is best to have it installed before the flowering stage commences. I recommend starting with a simple bamboo or wooden stake early in the vegetative stage and then, as the plant grows, you will be better informed to make a decision on what the next best level of support will be for your individual plant.

Shade for Your Plants

If the sun is too intense for your plants, you will see the top leaves begin to curl inward in an attempt to protect themselves from the sun's rays. You may also notice the leaves bleaching. This is more of a concern when your plants are young and small. It is especially important to shelter them from the sun when you are hardening them off (see page 121). As your plants get older and grow bigger, it is less important to provide them with shade from the sun.

If your plants are in pots, your best option is to move them to a shady area during the hottest part of the day (from noon until 3–4 p.m. or so). If your plants are planted in the ground, you can put four posts (made from wood, metal, or bamboo) around the perimeter of your plants, and then drape a shade cloth, a piece of burlap, or a light-colored, thin bedsheet on top to provide some sun protection.

With all this said, it is fairly rare for excessive sun to be an issue, but, depending on where you live and what the future effects of climate change are, shading plants may become a more common practice. I have found that, once your plants are in the ground and growing vigorously, they can quite easily handle the intense heat and rays of the sun and will thrive on those days.

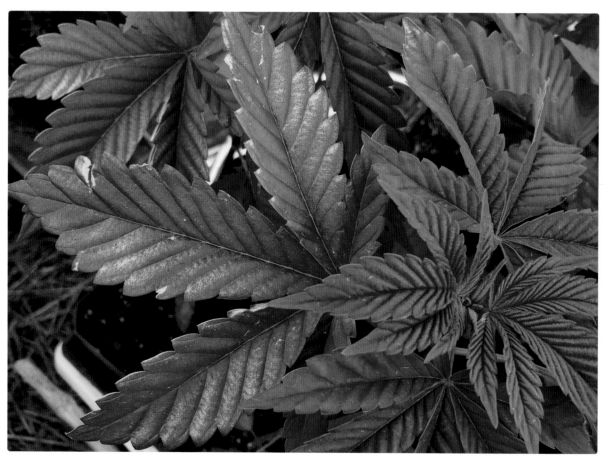

The leaves on the left show signs of bleaching, an indication of sunburn. Plants that have been grown indoors can be susceptible to sunburn if they have not been acclimated to the intensity of the sunlight through hardening.

FAQS & TROUBLESHOOTING

Q: What do I do if the water is running straight through my pots and the soil medium does not seem to be absorbing it?

A: This happens sometimes, especially when you're using a peat-based medium. You can try using a wetting agent, such as one made from yucca. Another trick is to place your pots in a tray and let your plants sit in the excess water for 20–30 minutes. They will draw up some of that water through the drainage holes in the pot and absorb it into the soil. Just make sure you do not leave them in the water too long.

Q: What is flushing? Do I need to flush my plants?

A: *Flushing* is a term used for running excess water without nutrients or fertilizers through your growing medium (and out the bottom of your pots). It is often done during the last two weeks of flowering or if you have used too much fertilizer, especially salt-based, synthetic fertilizers. It is important to wash or "flush" out the excess nutrients, as they will have a negative effect on the taste and the way your cannabis burns if used for smoking or vaping. When using living soils and amendments, you do not need to flush your plants.

Q: What are the signs of overwatering? What do I do if I've overwatered my plants?

A: Yellowing plant leaves and a droopy appearance can be signs of overwatering, along with soggy, poorly drained soil. If you suspect you have overwatered, make sure to let the soil dry out before watering again. If it is a pot that has been overwatered, make sure the air can freely circulate over the surface of the soil (you can use a fan for this) and maintain a warm, as opposed to a cool, environment whenever possible. When the pot has dried out, slowly water it again, making sure not to give it too much water. For your plants in the ground, they should be fine as long as you have well-drained soil. If you live in a very wet area with poor-draining soil, you should consider adding amendments, such as sand, to help prevent your plants from getting waterlogged with excessive rain.

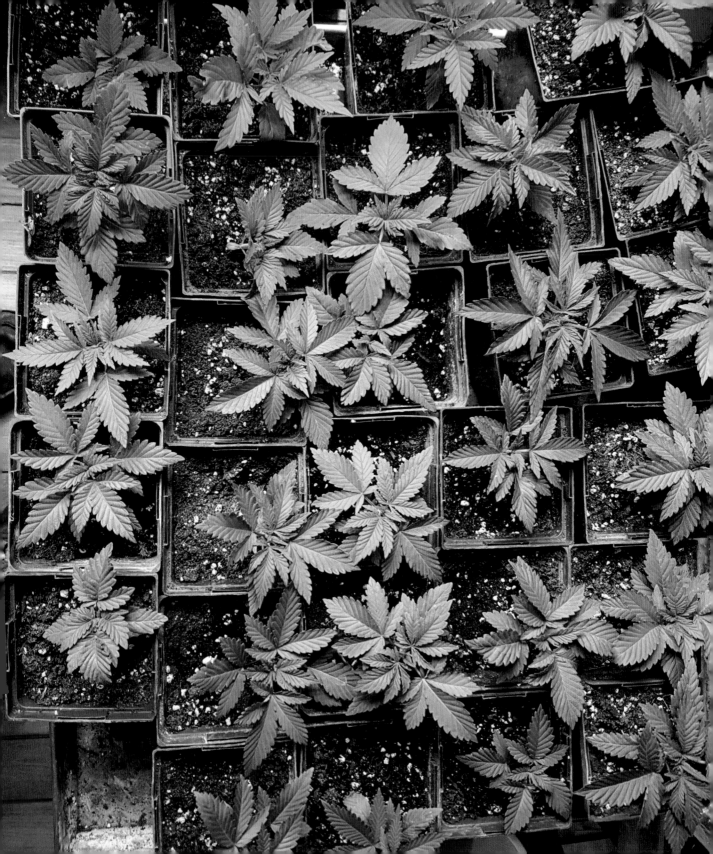

CHAPTER 7

< Seeds, Clones & Germination >

Many gardeners enjoy the annual ritual of looking through seed catalogs during the winter months—dreaming, planning, and envisioning all the plants they will grow in their gardens over the coming season. Cannabis growers do the same. They are constantly on the lookout for new cultivars and follow their favorite breeders in anticipation of growing a new plant in their gardens. Germinating seeds is exciting for any grower, but, for the beginner, it can also be a little daunting. This chapter will teach you how to select cultivars, choose seeds, and germinate them, as well as how to take your own cuttings and produce clones from mother plants.

HOW TO SELECT CULTIVARS

If you are new to cannabis, it can be overwhelming to look at the hundreds and even thousands of different cannabis varieties that are available. With names such as AK-47, Royal Sour Kush, Gorilla Glue #4, and Super Silver Haze, it can be hard to know where to start. To learn how to select the best cultivars for you, you need to think about your needs, look for high-quality genetics, and consider your growing conditions.

Considering Your Needs

One of the first and most important questions to ask yourself is this: What effects do you want to experience from using cannabis? Are you looking for a cultivar that uplifts or sedates? Is there a certain medical condition that you would like to address? Are you looking for a cultivar that is high in THC or CBD? How are you going to use the cannabis that you produce? Will you use it for smoking, vaping, hash or other concentrates, edibles, tinctures, salves, or oils? Once you know how you are planning to use your flowers, you can

LEFT These cannabis seedlings are three weeks old. In that time, they can grow to about 6 inches (15 cm) tall or more and have 3–5 sets of leaves.

< 107 >

then move onto selecting a cultivar that will meet your needs.

A commonly held belief is that indica plants (or BLD cultivars) are more sedating, while sativa plants (or NLD cultivars) are more uplifting. Although this is sometimes the case, it does not ring true for most cultivars these days because almost all of today's cannabis varieties are hybrids. Research has shown that it is often the terpenes in the trichomes, working synergistically with cannabinoids, that regulate or produce many of the effects that are commonly attributed solely to indica or sativa plants. For instance, myrcene, one of the most common terpenes in modern cannabis, is partly responsible for the sedating effects that are felt by the consumer and is also a muscle relaxant, pain reliever, and anti-inflammatory. On the other hand, limonene, which is often found in NLD cultivars, can produce uplifting or euphoric effects, and give people more motivation without leaving them feeling drained or burned out. Rather than focusing on the distinction between sativa and indica plants, I encourage you to do a little research on terpenes (the sidebar below will help you get started). You will begin to see some connection between the effects of certain cultivars and their terpene content.

COMMON TERPENES

Terpenes are responsible for the many beautiful aromas of the cannabis plant. More than two hundred terpenes have been identified in cannabis, but only about thirty are found in levels significant enough to have a therapeutic effect. Terpenes have many medicinal qualities and work synergistically with cannabinoids. Terpenes make up most of the essential oils of the plant and play a big role in the various medicinal effects of different cultivars.

Beta-Caryophyllene: Beta-caryophyllene is a common terpene that is also found in black pepper, cloves, and cinnamon. It has a sweet, woody aroma and is known to interact with CB2 receptors in the endocannabinoid system. Beta-caryophyllene is strongly anti-inflammatory and helps regulate the immune system. It can also be used as an analgesic and has antibacterial, antidepressant, anti-seizure, anti-spasmodic, and antioxidant properties.

Humulene: Humulene is a terpene with anti-inflammatory, antibacterial, anti-tumor, and analgesic properties. It has been used successfully as an appetite suppressant. It has a spicy, earthy, and woodsy aroma and is also found in cloves, hops, and basil.

Limonene: Limonene is what gives lemons their distinctive smell and is found in all citrus fruit. It is an immunostimulant and has antibacterial, antifungal, antidepressant, and anticonvulsive properties. Its antidepressive and euphoric effects are responsible for some varieties of cannabis that have uplifting effects.

Linalool: Linalool is responsible for a cultivar's calming, anti-anxiety effect. It is also an analgesic and acts as a sedative that can help you fall asleep. Lavender is another plant that contains linalool and has similar qualities; linalool is responsible for lavender's floral scent.

Myrcene: Myrcene is one of the most common terpenes in modern cannabis. It is an analgesic, and acts as a muscle relaxant and sedative. When combined with CBD, it helps to lower inflammation in the body. It is also found in mango and hops.

Ocimene: Ocimene has a very sweet and fruity aroma. It is not too stimulating nor too sedating, falling right in the middle of these two ends of the spectrum. It is antifungal, anticonvulsive, and anti-tumor.

Pinene: Alpha and beta pinene are found in coniferous trees, especially the pines trees (*Pinus* spp.). It acts as a bronchial dilator, inhibits cancer cell growth, and has anti-inflammatory and antibiotic properties. Uplifting in its effects, it can also increase your energy levels and level of concentration.

Terpinolene: Terpinolene is known to be uplifting and stimulating in its effect. It has a citrusy aroma and can provide cognitive clarity. It is antibacterial, antifungal, and anti-proliferative. It can inhibit cancer cell growth, and works as an antioxidant and sedative. In addition to cannabis, it is found in apple, cumin, lemon, and lilac.

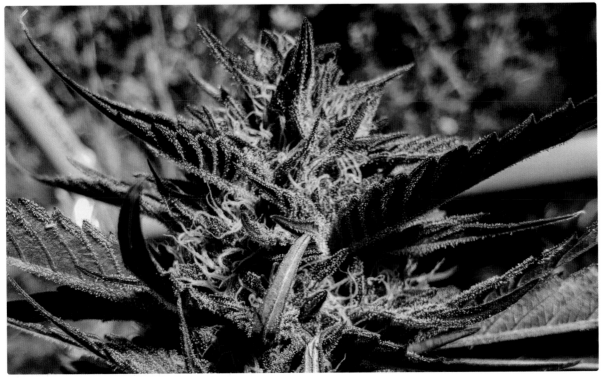

The Lavender Royal, shown here, is an example of a cultivar with great genetics. It produces compact, mold- and pest-resistant flowers that have a beautiful lavender smell with an earthy, spicy funk.

Each cultivar will also vary in terms of its cannabinoid levels, especially levels of CBD and THC. If you are looking to use cannabis medicinally for non-cancer-related therapy, research has shown that a 1:1 ratio between THC and CBD is often the most effective. Others may want a high-THC variety to treat pain, help with sleep, decrease stress, promote relaxation, stimulate appetite, and provide a host of other benefits. People often seek out cultivars high in CBD if they are not looking for the "high" that THC produces and want help with anxiety, localized pain relief, seizures, muscle spasms, and many other conditions.

TIP: Although there are many breeders selling seeds of high-CBD cultivars, it is important to note that not every seed is going to grow into a plant that produces flowers with high CBD content. It can take many years to stabilize a cultivar to the point where it always has the desired chemical constituents, and, unfortunately, some breeders will sell seeds that are not tested or fully developed or stabilized.

The Importance of Genetics

One of the most important things to consider when purchasing seeds or clones is their genetics.

The genetics of your seeds or clones affect the quality of your plants and their flowers. No matter how you take care of your plants, inferior genetics will never produce top-quality flowers, whereas quality genetics can often yield great results even with an inexperienced grower at the helm.

The marketplace for cannabis seeds has seen a huge influx of breeders in the last few years. Although there are many newer breeders who are releasing quality seeds, there are also many who are simply crossing one plant to another, coming up with a fancy-sounding name, and charging a lot of money for seeds and plants that have never really been tested. Reputable breeders will always test their seeds multiple times, making sure to select for strong, healthy plants that have high yields, produce buds with the desired potency, and are disease- or pest-resistant, among other characteristics. This type of time, work, and dedication creates high-quality genetics.

When you're making your first purchase, it is a good idea to look for seeds from established breeders who have been in the industry for a number of years and carry some older or unique cultivars, as opposed to new breeders pushing trendy strains. It is helpful to consider where the breeder is located as well. A breeder growing in California or Holland is more likely to have cultivars that do better in those regions than a breeder based in the Canadian Prairies. This is especially true when looking for cultivars that you plan to grow outdoors.

Considering Your Growing Environment

If you are looking to grow indoors, the possibilities are really endless. You can take (almost) complete control over the growing environment, meaning that selecting a cultivar to grow has less to do with the bioregion in which you live and more to do with your personal needs and preferences.

When it comes to growing outdoors, most cultivars will do well in a sunny southern region. If you live in the United States (especially the southern half of the country), you will be able to grow more varieties of cannabis because of the warmer climate and the longer growing season. If you live in the northern United States or Canada, you will have fewer options because the growing season is shorter. Most modern varieties have been bred to be grown indoors, and many of these cultivars will not do well in a cold, northern climate (or a moist, humid climate for that matter). But do not let this discourage you.

You will still be able to grow some top-quality cannabis, provided that you pick cultivars that can adapt to your specific area, growing season, and conditions. Look for hardier cultivars that have been proven to grow in your environment or autoflower cultivars if you do not live in a warm, sunny, southern region. These hardier varieties will be quick to finish; can handle the shorter, colder season; and are potentially mold- and disease-resistant. Most seed banks and breeders will include information about these characteristics on their website, in their catalog, or on the back of the seed packet. You can also go online or look in books and magazines to do your own research and find stories from other growers speaking about their personal experience with a specific cultivar.

To figure out which cultivars are best for your bioregion, ask yourself the following questions:

1. **How long is your growing season? In other words, how many consecutive frost-free days do you see in a year?** For example, here in the Great Lakes region, where I live, we are generally safe from frost between May 24 and the end of September, give or take a week or so on each side of the season. This gives us roughly 3½–4 months (though 4 months may be wishful thinking!) of a frost-free growing season.

2. **How much sunlight does your area get throughout the growing season and in the specific location where you are planting your plants?** You want your plants to have at least 6 hours of direct sunlight each day, preferably more.

3. **What are the weather conditions in your region and in the vicinity of your garden?** You'll want to note average temperature during the night and day, prevailing winds, frequency of precipitation, and the first and last frost days.

4. **During the growing season, what are the temperatures and humidity levels like in your area, and do they change between the start and the end of the season?** You need to determine whether you live in an environment that is moist and hot, cool and dry, hot and dry, or cold and wet.

Your answer to the last question will especially influence your choice of cultivar. If the weather in your area tends to be cool and humid, especially in the fall, you will want cultivars that are resistant to mold and powdery mildew, and finish early. Flowers that grow densely are more susceptible to botrytis (see page 215), especially in wet climates. If you are in a colder environment, you will want to look for varieties that are more cold-tolerant. If you are in a warm and dry habitat with a long growing season, you may want to try some varieties that have a longer growing cycle or plants that produce large, dense flowers.

These guidelines are by no means an exhaustive list, but they offer a helpful place to start. From here, your experience growing will be the best thing to guide you moving forward. Each year, you will learn more and be able to try cultivars with different genetics or even breed your own cultivars (see page 157 for more information on breeding).

HOW TO SELECT SEEDS

Cannabis seeds are sold in small packages containing a specific number of seeds, usually between six and twelve seeds per package. Stored in the right conditions (see page 161), they will stay viable for a number of years, so you do not have to worry about planting them all at once. Cannabis seeds can be very expensive. The price of one seed can range from a couple of dollars to $25 or more. Consider them as an investment, especially when there is the potential for each seed to grow into plants that produce many flowers.

All seeds sold by reputable breeders should have close to a 100 percent germination rate, but there are several variables that will affect whether your seeds will germinate, such as how deep you plant them, temperature and humidity levels, and the composition of the soil. With optimal conditions and quality seeds, you can expect to have 80–100 percent of your seeds sprout.

The number of seeds you plant will be dictated by the number of plants you are legally able to grow. You may also have personal goals and constraints that affect the number of plants that you can care for. Make sure you know how many plants you can legally grow, and plant your seeds accordingly. It's not a bad idea to start small.

Where to Find Seeds

You have a number of choices when looking for a place to obtain seeds:

- **Licensed retailers:** There may be licensed distributors or retailers in your state or province that sell seeds. This can be a good place to start because these companies are sanctioned and regulated by the government.

- **Cannabis conventions, trade shows, or festivals:** These events often have breeders and seed companies that will set up booths to sell their seeds.

- **Seed banks:** You can find seed banks that will carry a number of different cultivars from many breeders online. Try to purchase from ones that have a good reputation, have positive reviews, and are known to test the genetic stability of their cultivars.

- **Friends and neighbors:** There may be local growers or you might have friends in your area who have extra seeds to donate, trade, or sell. As time goes by, this option will become available to more people. It is my hope that cannabis seeds will one day be traded back and forth, just as tomato or other vegetable seeds are often shared among friends.

When obtaining seeds, it is important to check the laws of your state or province, and country before making a purchase, especially if you're purchasing seeds through the mail. In many countries, it is legal to sell cannabis seeds as "souvenirs," as the seeds do not contain any THC or CBD. The laws vary from location to location, so be sure to do your research and use your own discretion.

Types of Seeds

When you're ready to buy seeds, you'll find that you have a few different options. There are three types of seeds that are popular with home growers. The type that you choose will depend on your personal preference and your available growing conditions.

Regular Seeds

Regular seeds contain the genetics from both the male and female parents. Once sprouted, a seed will develop into either a male or female plant. In most cases, you will have a 50/50 chance of getting a male or female plant from a regular seed. For many people, especially those who plan to breed, these seeds are your best option.

Feminized Seeds

Feminized seeds are seeds that produce female plants (with very few exceptions). Breeders produce feminized seeds by stressing a female plant. This causes it to produce male flowers that pollinate its female flowers, which produces female plants in the next generation. Be aware that some methods of feminizing seeds involve the use of toxic chemicals, which is not environmentally friendly or sustainable. However, feminized seeds can be a good option for the home grower, especially if you live in a province or state that limits the number of plants in your home. You will not

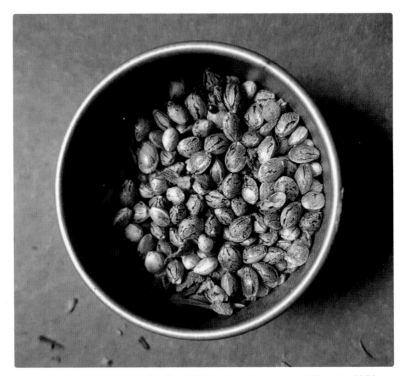

This container holds regular seeds for a high-CBD plant that I've bred myself. There is a 50/50 chance for each of these seeds to grow into a female plant. The presence of black "tiger" stripes means that the seeds are mature.

need to plant extra seeds to make up for any male plants that will have to be culled later to maximize your harvest.

Autoflower Seeds

Autoflower seeds will produce plants that are not photoperiod-dependent. Cannabis begins flowering as the hours of daylight decrease within a twenty-four-hour period; this occurs when summer turns to autumn. Autoflower plants will automatically begin to flower after a very short vegetative stage, even in the long days of summer, going from seed to harvest in 55–100 days, depending on the specific cultivar. These seeds are produced by crossing or breeding a cultivar that flowers normally with *Cannabis ruderalis*. Autoflower cultivars, known as "autos," have improved tremendously over the last decade. These seeds can be good options for growers who live in a northern climate, where the growing season is short, or for people who would like smaller, easier-to-grow plants. They could also be a good option for people who would like to get multiple harvests throughout one growing season, which can be done by doing successive plantings of autoflower seeds.

GERMINATING SEEDS

The two most common ways to germinate seeds are using a paper towel for the initial germination (see page 116) or planting the seeds directly into soil in a cell pack, pot, or the ground (see page 116). Both methods work well. Planting seeds directly into your outdoor cannabis beds, after the last frost, can also be a great option, especially if you live in a warmer climate. Whatever method you choose, remember to keep the soil or paper towel moist to aid the germination process.

Fresh and viable seeds should crack and sprout within a couple of days. It may take another couple of days for the sprout to grow a small root or breach the surface of the soil. If you plant seeds into soil, you should see the plants rising above its horizon between 3 and 7 days. Older seeds will take longer to emerge. They may need up to 14 days to sprout, so be patient and give them some time before you give up hope.

If you are growing indoors, you can start the germination process at any time you wish. If you are germinating seeds to plant outdoors, I recommend that you begin the process approximately 4–6 weeks before it is safe to plant outside and the risk of frost and cold temperatures has passed. For example, if May 24 marks the beginning of outdoor planting time in your area, you should plant your seeds between April 12 and 26. In some areas of the United States, it may be possible to plant your seeds directly into the ground in your garden beds. But, in most places, it is better to start your seeds indoors or in a greenhouse before moving them outdoors and then eventually transplanting them into the ground.

When starting your seeds in cell packs or small pots, be sure to use a light potting soil. With a light potting soil, the seeds will not have to use more of their energy reserves to emerge from the ground.

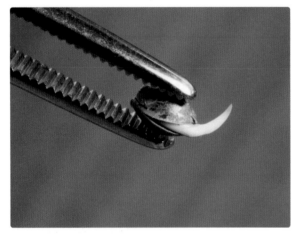

You can use tweezers to pick up seeds that have sprouted, as long as you avoid damaging the radicle, or embryonic root of the plant.

Paper Towel Method

1. Place the seeds in a small glass of nonchlorinated water.

2. Let the seeds sit overnight or 18–24 hours. They should sink after a couple of hours. You can poke them with your finger to facilitate sinking. Fresh seeds will begin to crack in as little as a few hours, while older seeds will be slower and should be soaked for an extra 24 hours. If your seeds crack open, you can move onto the next step. If not, wait the additional 24 hours.

3. After soaking, place the seeds in a folded, wet paper towel, and set the paper towel on a plate. Put the plate in a warm place, such as on a heating pad, on top of a fridge, in a warmer spot in your house, or under a humidity dome.

4. Wait for your seeds to sprout. If the seeds are fresh, they should do so within a couple of days. Older seeds will take longer—1 week, sometimes up to 2 weeks. Be sure to keep the paper towel moist throughout this time, using a spray bottle.

5. Once the roots are ¼–½ inch (6–13 mm) long, they are ready to be planted in the soil. Follow steps 1–4 below to complete your planting.

Direct Planting into Soil

1. Water the soil before you plant your seeds. By doing this, you do not disturb the seed by watering it after it has been planted.

2. Poke a little hole in the soil with a pen or pencil. The depth of this hole should be approximately twice the width of the seed.

3. Place the seed into the hole with the pointy end (with the root, if it has sprouted) down. Cover the seed gently with soil. Once the seed is planted, you can use a spray bottle filled with water to moisten the top layer of soil.

4. Repeat steps 1–3 for each seed that you want to plant.

5. After planting your seeds, you can leave them in the dark and move them to a location with proper lighting after they begin to sprout and grow above the horizon line of the soil. Your seedlings should emerge within 2–7 days. Fresh, healthy seeds should break the soil horizon fairly quickly, while older seeds may take a little longer. Keep the soil moist, but not sopping wet, and have some patience.

EARLY SEEDLING CARE

This early stage of your plant's life is an exciting time. You have witnessed the magic of the seed germinating and sprouting, and now you have a little plant to take care of. Your plants will have enough stored energy to grow without any added nutrients for the next couple of weeks, but you still need to make sure you provide the right environment for them to grow strong and healthy. This is especially important at this initial stage of your plants' lives. Added stress during this time may negatively affect the growth and health of your plants now and can set them back. These are your babies—nurture them and treat them right, and they will repay you tenfold come harvest time.

Lighting

It is important to give seedlings adequate light, either from indoor grow lights or the sun outside, as soon as they begin to emerge. Otherwise, they will begin to "stretch" and become leggy, developing long stems that make the plant weaker and susceptible to falling over.

If you are relying on the sun in the early spring, especially at northern latitudes, your plants may not get enough light throughout the day. They may begin to flower early as a result, leading to a very limited yield and wasting your time, money, and energy. You will need to add supplemental lighting to keep your plants in the vegetative state. This supplemental lighting can be as simple as placing your plants in a room and leaving the light on for four or five hours after the sun goes down. You can also set up a small lamp, a fluorescent light, or a grow light above your plants for these extra hours.

Make sure to pay attention to the placement of your grow lights. If you're using fluorescent grow lights, you can keep them close to the tops of your plants. If you're using other lights, such as LED or HID lighting, be sure to place them farther away. Otherwise, you run the risk of giving your seedlings too much light and "burning" them. Your light cycle should be set on timers that turn your lights on for 18 hours and shut them off for 6 hours during each 24-hour period to avoid early flowering.

Growing Conditions

You want to make sure your growing environment is consistently warm (72–76°F [22–24°C]) and has stable humidity levels (around 50–60 percent). If you've planted your seeds in containers, you may want to use a heat mat to keep the soil and the roots of your young seedlings a few degrees warmer than the ambient air temperature. This is not necessary, but it can be a good idea if your growing environment is on the cooler side or has fluctuations in temperature. The extra warmth will promote healthy root growth.

Watering

It is very important not to overwater or overfertilize your young plants. Your plant is small at this time and has a very small root system. It does not have the ability to absorb an overabundance of water, nor does it need so much water. It is best

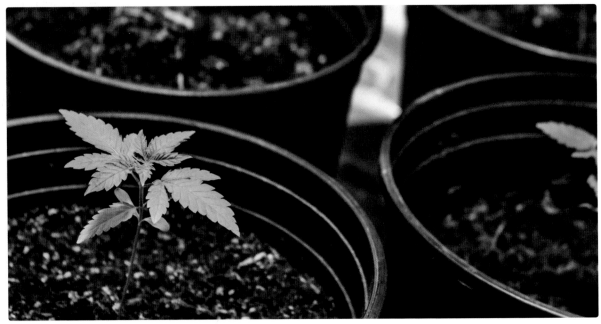

It is important to avoid growing young plants in containers that are too big. A properly sized container will prevent problems with overwatering and make plants more forgiving of the mistakes of inexperienced growers.

to let your cell packs or pots begin to dry out between waterings.

Nutrition

Once your plants grow approximately 7–8 inches (18–20 cm) tall and have multiple sets of leaves, you may want to give them a little fertilizer. An easy way to tell if your plant could use more nutrients is by observing its color. Vibrant green plants that do not show any signs of yellowing do not need any fertilizer. A plant that starts to change color could benefit from a light feeding (check out chapter 13 for more on deficiencies).

When adding nutrients, be very careful and only apply diluted amounts. Young seedlings do not need a lot of nutrients, so you want to make sure that you do not feed your plants more than they can handle. If you are mixing a potting soil,

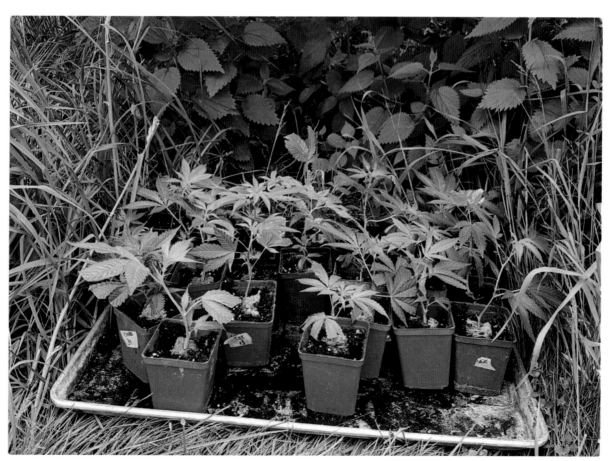

These cuttings have been placed outside to harden off (and can also benefit from a light feeding of fertilizer). After experiencing a couple inches of new growth, they will be ready to be planted into the ground.

be sure not to add too many soil amendments. If you are purchasing a growing medium, check the label to see if it is "charged," which means fertilizer has been added. For bottled nutrients, be sure to only give your plants a quarter of the strength recommended on the label.

Transplanting

After a few weeks, you will notice your plants really starting to take off. There will be a lot of new growth from the leaf and stem nodes and an uptick in vertical growth as they begin to enter the vegetative growth stage. We will talk more about this stage in the next chapter.

In the meantime, you may need to transplant your seedling into a bigger pot (see page 98). You do not want your plant to become root-bound, which slows growth and sometimes impairs its ability to take up the nutrients necessary to maintain health.

When you transplant, you will want to mix up a new batch of soil that contains organic amendments and a good mix of organic material. I recommend transplanting seedlings from a cell pack to a 4-inch (10-cm) wide pot and then into a 1-gallon (3.8-L) pot. Once they are growing vigorously and have doubled in size in a 1-gallon pot, you can then transplant them outside or into the pot that they will stay in for the remainder of their life.

If you are growing outdoors, your young plant is ready to be moved directly into the ground for the rest of the season after it has grown about 1–2 feet (30–61 cm) tall. It will be safe to plant young plants in the ground after the last frost and once they have been hardened off. Research your local weather patterns and do your best to estimate when the last frost will be. If you have never grown plants outside before, ask a local gardener when they plant their tomatoes or peppers in the ground. Their answer will give you a good idea about when it is safe to plant your cannabis as well. Be sure to take about a week or so to harden your plants off to outdoor conditions (see page 121) before planting them in the ground or exposing them to the direct intensity of the sun for an entire day.

I suggest digging as big of a hole as possible for each cannabis plant, about 3 feet (91 cm) wide and deep, and amending the soil by adding inputs into the hole before planting your cannabis in the ground. Space out your plants 8–10 feet (2.4–3 m) apart from each other, measuring the center of one hole to the center of the next one. Cannabis is a heavy feeder, meaning it requires a lot of nutrients from the soil to flourish and grow dense, heavy flowers. To make sure it has the nutrients it needs, try using the soil mixes described on page 82. If you are confident that your garden bed is well amended and full of healthy living soil, you can dig a small hole just big enough to put your plant into. The choice is yours.

HARDENING OFF

Hardening off your plants refers to acclimatizing them to the elements. This is a very important step, especially when moving young indoor plants to the outdoors. You do not want to expose plants grown under artificial lights to prolonged direct sunlight right away. The light is too powerful for your plants at this time and can potentially burn them, similar to how some people's skin may initially be prone to sunburn after a winter of being covered up.

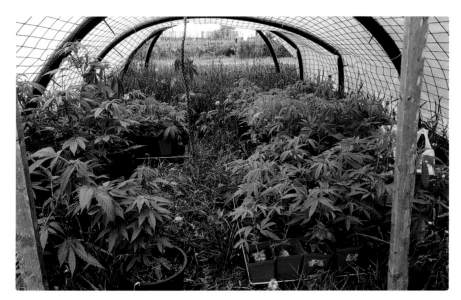

This hoop house, made from an old chicken tractor and a white tarp, has been repurposed to create a hardening area. The tarp diffuses the intensity of the sunlight to allow the plants to acclimatize to outdoor conditions and protects them from the elements. You can also simply place your plants in a shady spot under a tree and out of the wind to harden your plants.

You first want to move your plants to a shady location where they receive dappled light and no more than a couple of hours of direct sunlight each day. Over the course of a week or so, you can slowly increase the amount of direct sunlight that they receive daily, and after this period of time, they will be ready for full days of direct sunlight. Always keep an eye on your plants during this process, and make sure that the leaves stay dark green. Leaves that have faded to yellow are a sign of burning. Leaves that are curling and closing in on themselves can be a sign of too much sun as well.

Your plants also need to harden off to the other elements, such as wind, rain, hail, and more. Be sure that your plants are well supported with stakes (if needed) and are not falling over. Because they are not used to strong winds or rain at this point, make sure to place the plants in a spot that protects them from these forces of nature. In general, after 7–10 days, your plants should acclimate to their new environment and be ready for rapid growth.

CLONES

Clones are cuttings taken from another cannabis plant. Cloning is an easy way to produce plants that will be genetically the same as the mother plant (the plant from which you take cuttings). It lets you propagate cannabis quickly and efficiently; allows you to grow a garden where all the plants have uniform growth, potency, and harvest times; and does not require you to wait for a seed to sprout or determine the sex of your plants.

Selecting a Mother Plant

A good mother plant candidate is a plant with your desired traits (such as medicinal properties, taste, smell, pest- or disease-resistance, yield, or genetic stability). Mother plants are typically grown from seed and kept in a vegetative state. It is best to wait until they are approximately 2 months old before taking cuttings. If you take your cuttings too early, it can stunt their growth.

Mother plants can be kept in a vegetative state for years as long as you can take them inside, provide them with 18 hours of light (preferably from metal halide or LED lights), and avoid overfeeding them. Growers will often give mother plants 10 percent less nitrogen than what is usually recommended; this helps them avoid growing too quickly and allows the clones to root faster.

You can easily take thousands and thousands of clones from a healthy mother plant kept in the vegetative state. Some people choose to take cuttings from a healthy, outdoor plant before it enters the flowering stage. By doing this, you can use this cutting to "preserve" the mother plant through the winter season by growing the clone indoors. You can then take additional cuttings from the clone for the next outdoor season or use it in various breeding projects. There are a lot of possibilities!

Eventually, you will need to replace a mother plant—you can either clone the mother plant to create the replacement, bring in a clone of another plant, or start with a new plant grown from seed. It is very important to keep an eye on your mother plants for any signs of disease, fungal infection, or pests. If your mother plants become infected by disease or fungi, they will pass it onto the clones. It is often best to discard a diseased plant and start over again.

How to Create Clones

To clone a plant, you should cut a branch off the mother plant and encourage the cutting to grow roots by placing it in a rooting medium. A rooting medium can be the soil that you use to fill your pots, or you can use popular materials, such as rockwool, peat pucks, coco coir, sand, or premade soil mixes. It is important for the rooting medium to be lofty or airy, remain moist but not too wet, and stay warm. Some of these materials are more sustainable than others, and it is up to you to use what you feel comfortable using and supporting.

You will also find rooting hormone to be helpful. Using either a homemade or store-bought rooting hormone will decrease the time it takes your clones to develop roots and increase your overall success rate. Store-bought products can come in powder or gel form.

It is best to root your cuttings indoors or in a greenhouse where you can monitor and maintain a consistent environment. Keeping your cannabis cutting warm at a high humidity level (approximately 75°F [24°C] and 80–85 percent humidity) will allow it to root more quickly and produce strong and vibrant plants. Propagation trays along with clear humidity domes and a heat mat for cool environments will help maintain the proper conditions.

You may be able to purchase clones from a licensed nursery. Make sure that they come from a trusted source, were grown in a clean environment, and have not come into contact with any pests or disease. Be sure to carefully inspect any plants you pick up and

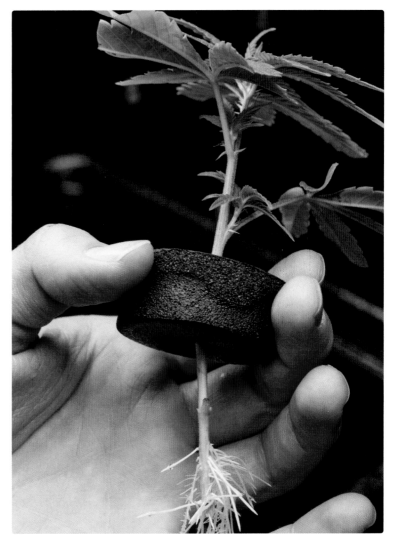

After a clone has grown roots, it can be transplanted into a pot or planted directly into the ground if you live in a warm climate or there is no danger of frost. Once the root system is established, you will begin to notice rapid vertical growth.

do not introduce them into your growing environment until you are sure they are healthy. The last thing you want to do is bring into your garden or grow room an unhealthy plant that infects the rest of your plants.

Steps to Successful Cloning

What You Need

Pitcher or cup for holding cuttings

Bowl

Water*

Scissors

Razor blade

Rooting hormone of your choice,
   store-bought or homemade

Rooting medium of your choice
   (see page 122 for options)**

Humidity dome

Cell packs, one for each clone (if needed for
   your chosen rooting medium), and
   propagation tray

Heating mat (optional)

Thermometer hygrometer

*It is ideal to use nonchlorinated water with a pH between 6.0 and 6.5.

**If using rockwool cubes, they should be presoaked in water with a pH of 5.5.

> **TIP:** Make sure you have all the tools you need beforehand and sanitize your cutting implements. Isopropyl alcohol works well for keeping blades clean.

1. Fill the pitcher or cup and the bowl with nonchlorinated water.

2. Choose a branch or growing tip from your mother plant that has at least three sets of leaves on it. Using a pair of scissors, cut off this branch and place it into the pitcher or cup of water. You can place multiple cuttings into the same pitcher or cup of water.

3. Take off the bottom set of leaves on each cutting. If a cutting has large leaves, you may want to give it a "haircut" by trimming half the tips off each leaf.

4. With a razor blade, make a second cut at a 45-degree angle, just below a node (the place where the leaf meets the stem). Leave the node on the cutting. I always make this second cut in a bowl of water, with the cut end slightly submerged. Doing this allows the cut end to come into immediate contact with water, limiting the chance of an air embolism entering the stem of the new plant.

5. Dip the cut end into the rooting hormone of your choice. For example, you can use a homemade willow bark tea (see page 102 for a recipe) as a natural rooting agent or make the Natural Rooting Hormone Paste, using the recipe on page 126.

6. Insert your cutting into your rooting medium of choice in a propagation tray, making sure the medium holds it firmly in place and it stays upright.

7. Repeat steps 1–6 for any additional cuttings that you want to take.

8. When you have taken all the cuttings you need, place a humidity dome on top of the propagation tray and set the tray under the light of your

choice (be careful not to place them too close to powerful lights). If your space is on the cooler side, place the tray on top of a heating mat, if desired. Clones need 18 hours of light per 24-hour cycle. Fluorescent lights and other similar low-wattage lights work great for rooting cuttings.

9. For the first two days, keep the humidity close to 100 percent, using a thermometer hygrometer to check. On the third day, start opening the vent holes of the humidity dome slightly to decrease the humidity to around 80 percent. It is also a good idea to take your domes off the tray once a day for 30 seconds to one minute to exchange all the air inside the dome. After one week, you can decrease the humidity to 65–70 percent. If your plants start to wilt, close the vent holes and let the humidity rise a little.

10. Between 10 days and 2 weeks later, you should start to see roots coming out of the bottom of your rooting medium. Once there are a number of roots showing, your clones are ready to be transplanted into pots.

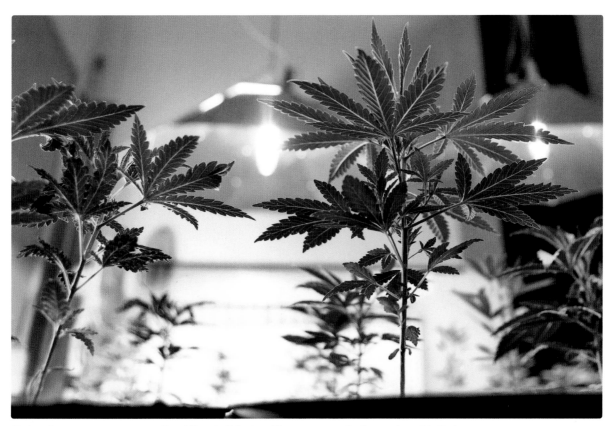

Cloning allows you to propagate cannabis quickly and efficiently and is a common practice in nurseries and for the home grower.

Natural Rooting Hormone Paste

Willow bark is a great natural root enhancer that contains two auxins, hormones that regulate growth: salicylic acid and indolebutyric acid. The aloe gel helps the paste adhere to the stem of the cutting, and it contains many vitamins, enzymes, and amino acids, and is a source of salicylic acid as well. This recipe may make more paste than you need. Only mix up what you will use. You can freeze extra willow water and aloe separately in ice cube trays. Before using again, defrost the water and aloe and then mix them together just before use.

What You Need

Small willow tree branch (from any member of the genus *Salix* spp.)

Water

1 piece of aloe vera, about 3–6 inches (7.5–15 cm) long

1. Follow steps 1–4 of the Willow Bark Tea recipe (page 102).

2. After the willow bark tea has steeped overnight, strain the tea.

3. Scrape out gel from the aloe vera and put in a small cup or bowl.

4. Mix about a ¼ cup (60 ml) of the willow bark tea and aloe together to form a paste or a mixture with a milkshake consistency. Dip your cuttings into the paste.

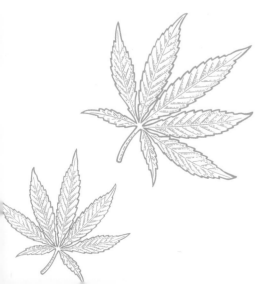
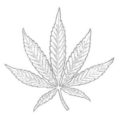
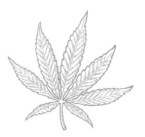

FAQS & TROUBLESHOOTING

Q: Is it worth it to pay so much money for cannabis seeds?

A: Cannabis seeds are sometimes not worth the prices that some people charge, especially when one plant can produce thousands and thousands of seeds. There are some breeders who should not be charging the prices they do, but, that said, there are also great breeders out there who put in a huge amount of time, effort, and passion into creating amazing cultivars and only release seeds that they stand behind. These breeders should be compensated for all they have invested in this process. If you want to avoid the steep prices altogether, I recommend that you become self-sufficient by producing your own seeds. (You will learn how to breed your plants in chapter 9.)

Q: How many seeds should I plant if I have regular seeds and want to have four females in total?

A: Because you never really know what the sex of your seeds is going to be, I recommend planting 6–8 seeds. It will generally take 4–6 weeks (sometimes longer) before they show signs of sex through their pre-flowers. If you end up with more females than you need, give one to a friend or neighbor, if it is legal to do so in your area.

Q: I have old seeds. What should I do if I want to try to germinate them?

A: The age of your seeds and the way they were stored will affect your germination rate. I recommend soaking your old seeds until they crack open. You can scarify the horizontal edge of the seeds with a small piece of 120-grit sandpaper. This will help the seed to open more easily. You can also make a seed treatment solution called SES, which is commonly used in Korean natural farming. You can find recipes for SES and other methods for encouraging germination online.

Q: Some of my seeds aren't sprouting. What happened?

A: It is hard to say for sure why your seeds did not sprout. Your seeds may have been immature and they may have been harvested before they were fully developed. They also could be old seeds that did not have enough energy reserves left to sprout. Environmental conditions could be a factor as well. For example, the temperature may have been too cold. If you have a germination rate of zero, something was likely wrong with the entire batch of seeds or some sort of environmental condition affected all the seeds at once. If you purchased these seeds from a breeder or a seed bank, I would reach out to them and let them know about your germination rate. They may refund your money or give you new seeds.

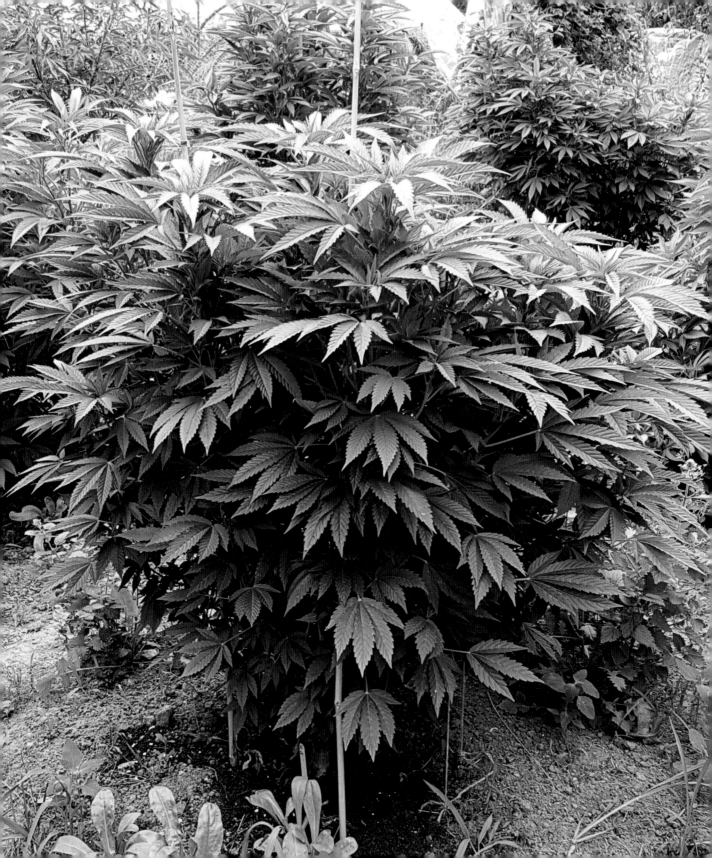

CHAPTER 8

< Vegetative Growth >

Although each stage of growth for the cannabis plant is exciting, there is something special about this one. The vegetative growth stage is when a healthy cannabis plant really takes off and experiences explosive growth, reaching and stretching toward the heavens. It is a time to revel in the beauty and strength of this plant and a time when it needs support, love, and care to reach its full potential. In this chapter we will begin to outline the skills, tools, and techniques that you can use to optimize growth, and how you as the grower can play a big role in helping your plants thrive.

SIGNS OF VEGETATIVE GROWTH

During the vegetative stage of growth, your young seedlings will grow into a large plant. Healthy plants can grow between 1 and 2 inches (2.5 and 5 cm) per day. You will see thicker and stronger stalks appear, which will support the heavy flowers that will come in the next stage of growth. You may be amazed at how quickly your plant increases in diameter as well. There are not many annual herbaceous plants that can put on as much growth, girth, and density as cannabis.

During the vegetative stage, your plant will also send roots out in search of nutrients and develop symbiotic relationships with bacteria and fungi in the soil. This allows it to create a healthy soil microbiome, which will ultimately help the plant become strong and healthy.

LEFT Vegetative growth is the stage in which you will see the most rapid growth in your cannabis plant both in terms of its height and its width. This plant has bamboo stakes for support. You can provide more support by adding a wire cage around it as it continues to grow.

< 129 >

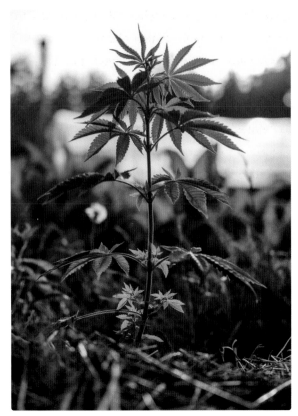

This young cannabis plant in the early stages of vegetative growth has just been planted in the ground. Once the roots are established in the soil, it will begin to grow quickly and vigorously toward the sun.

PLANT CARE FOR VEGETATIVE GROWTH

Providing a stable environment and the necessary nutrients is key to giving your plants the best conditions for growth and prevents any pests or disease from taking hold during this important stage.

Lighting

Most cannabis is photoperiod-dependent, so the amount of light it receives will determine how long the plant stays in the vegetative stage. When grown indoors, your plants will stay in a vegetative state indefinitely as long as you have your lights set to provide 18 hours of light and 6 hours of darkness. When grown outdoors, the plant will stay in the vegetative stage until the days begin to shorten and the amount of available sunlight decreases. In most areas, this happens around August 1, though it may occur earlier or later in the year, depending on your latitude.

Growing Conditions

For indoor plants, you want the temperature of your grow space to stay consistently warm (72°F–76°F [22°C–24°C]) with stable humidity (around 50–60 percent). When plants are grown outdoors, the temperature and humidity are outside your control. That said, you should always be aware of the average weather conditions during the spring and fall and plan your planting and harvesting times accordingly. Generally speaking, outdoor plants are a lot more resilient when it comes to temperature and humidity swings than plants grown in a controlled environment indoors.

Watering

Cannabis plants in vegetative growth require a lot of water, but be careful not to overdo it. Cannabis likes a well-drained soil. The root zone should not remain wet and soggy for a long period of time, and you should allow your plants to dry out between waterings, especially when you're growing them in pots. With outdoor plants growing in the ground, overwatering is less of a concern, but it still is something to be aware of. There is a better chance that the soil will drain excess water, and the roots will also be able to grow outward, making it unlikely that they will be sitting in soil that is constantly wet.

To avoid overwatering, make sure you are not watering your plants if the soil is already wet, it has just rained, or there is rain in the immediate forecast. For outdoor plants growing vigorously and not receiving any rainfall, you will need to water your plants once or twice per week. In some dry regions, you may have to water outdoor plants every 2–3 days. Plants growing outdoors in wetter regions may require significantly less watering.

Nutrition

During vegetative growth, your plants will be looking for and using a lot of nitrogen. As we outlined in the chapter on soil and nutrients, a well-balanced, healthy, living soil with an occasional addition of the proper organic amendments will have all the nutrients a plant needs.

If you do not have living soil or the time to build it, there are alternatives for ensuring that your plants have enough nutrients. I encourage you to try at least one or two of the nutrient sources and fertilizers listed in this section. You should begin fertilizing your plants after your plants have begun to grow vigorously and are

approximately 12–24 inches (30–61 cm) tall (it can be a little less for indoor plants).

I recommend that you give your plants additional nutrients about once every 1–2 weeks throughout the vegetative cycle and follow the guidelines listed in the recipes for homemade fertilizers. If you have not added any organic amendments to your soil previously, you will want to feed them more frequently. It is best to stop your vegetative fertilization program about 2 weeks before flowering begins. This will help your plants smoothly transition into this stage.

Alfalfa Pellets and Dried Alfalfa

Alfalfa provides many beneficial nutrients to your cannabis plants. It is a rich source of nitrogen and also contains phosphorus, potassium, sulfur, iron, and magnesium. Alfalfa comes in a few different forms. You can use fresh plant matter, dried plant material (such as alfalfa hay), or the alfalfa pellets commonly sold as a food for horses and rabbits at your local animal feed store or garden center. Just make sure that the pellets only contain alfalfa and avoid those with any other fillers or unnatural binding products.

You can apply alfalfa in pellet or plant form as a top dress for your soil, or you can use the plant matter and pellets to make a tea (see page 133 for a recipe). Some growers will choose to use alfalfa hay as mulch. Because alfalfa is high in nitrogen, it usually only needs to be applied twice during the vegetative stage when used as a top dress or tea.

Plant Teas

You can make teas from various plants, including alfalfa; red clover and other legumes; nettle; comfrey; horsetail; and other fast-growing, tall plants that are local to your region. These teas can be fermented (see recipe on page 133) and can be brewed using hot or cold water (I recommend cold water).

To source plant material for teas, you can pick plants that are growing wild in your area. If you are not familiar with the plants in your area, pick up a wildflower identification guide, such as *Newcomb's Wildflower Guide* by Lawrence Newcomb. Or, better yet, grow your desired plants in your garden and have direct access to them throughout the growing season.

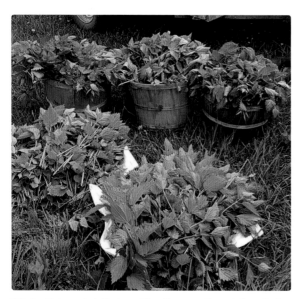

This freshly harvested stinging nettle will serve as the main ingredient for a large batch of plant tea.

GUIDELINES FOR FORAGING PLANTS FOR TEAS

- Always harvest from the point of view of a caretaker or land steward. Give thanks and gratitude for the plants, and do your best to leave the area better than you found it.

- Look for areas that are clean and free of chemical sprays, pollution, and signs of diseased or unhealthy plants. Stay away from roadsides, abandoned commercial or industrial areas, railway tracks, and areas under power lines—these places could contain contaminants and are often sprayed with chemical herbicides.

- Always be sure that you can identify the plant you are foraging with 100 percent certainty. This is important so that you can recognize it in the wild and find out if it can be sustainably harvested or not.

- Avoid harvesting any species that are rare, threatened, or endangered. Focus on gathering non-native species whenever possible.

- Only harvest what you need, and make sure that you use what you harvest and not let it go to waste. Always compost any excess plant material that you have harvested.

- Always make sure you have permission to harvest on the land that you are on and that you are following any laws or legal guidelines in place.

Fermented Plant Tea

Fermenting a plant tea involves extracting the nutrients out of the plants using water and a little sugar or molasses. Fermented plant teas are easy to make, low in cost, and a good way to add nutrition to and boost fertility in your garden. I recommend that you use the fresh plant for your teas whenever possible, but you can also make it with dried plant material if that is all that is available to you.

YIELD: 5 gallons (19 L)

What You Need

Plant material of your choice (see page 135 for suggestions), approximately 2½ gallons (9.5 L) or enough to fill a 5-gallon (19-L) bucket halfway

Water

1 cup (240 ml) molasses or brown sugar

Air pump or aerator (see page 24)

Tip: Chop up the plant material into 2–3-inch (5–7.5-cm) pieces to expose more surface area of the material to the water and sugar. This will also help you fit more plant material into the bucket.

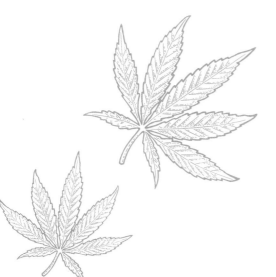

1. Fill half of a 5-gallon (19-L) bucket with plant material. Fill the remaining half of the bucket with water, making sure to cover all the plant material. It may take a while for the plant material to absorb the water and become submerged. After adding the water, let it rest for 2–3 hours and check back to see if you need to add more water. It is a good idea to put some kind of weight on top of the plant material to keep it submerged in the water. A plate, a rock, or a piece of wood works well for this purpose.

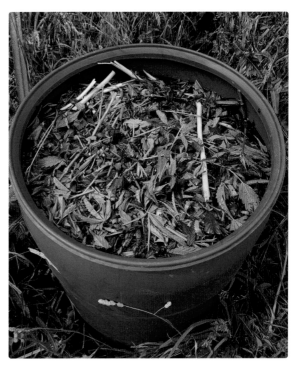

Plant teas can be made from a wide range of plants. This barrel is filled with leaves and stems from comfrey, stinging nettle, yarrow, and a male cannabis plant.

2. Add the molasses or brown sugar and stir to combine. Put the bucket in a shady spot. Be sure to cover it with a lid to avoid unwanted material or insects from getting into it.

3. Stir the solution a few times a day for 2–7 days. The time frame will be longer if temperatures are cold; less if they are hot. You want the water to change to a dark color and an almost sweet, fermented smell to emanate from the bucket. If it begins to smell unpleasant, this is a sign to strain it and move on to the next step. It is best to strain it before it begins to smell at all unpleasant.

4. Remove the plant material with a strainer so you are just left with liquid in the bucket. Add an air pump to the bucket to keep the mixture oxygenated and circulating in the bucket. Let the mixture bubble for 12–24 hours. The tea should still have a sweet scent, and you may also notice bubbles forming on the top of the water. This is a good sign.

5. To apply the tea when watering, mix 1 part tea to 5 parts water for soil watering. To use as a foliar spray (see page 68), mix 1 part tea and 10 parts water in a spray bottle. The color of the water will depend on the plants that are used to make the tea. Once it is diluted and ready for use, it will be lighter in color. The diluted solution can be used for watering or as a foliar spray once every 7–10 days during vegetative growth. It can also be mixed with compost and manure tea (see recipe on page 136.)

STORAGE: This tea should be used within 1–2 days after it has been brewed. If it is starting to smell unpleasant, that is a sign that it should be used right away before it spoils.

Tip: To brew an unfermented tea, just leave out the molasses mentioned in the recipe and only let it steep for 2 days before using.

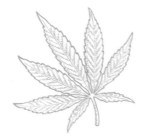

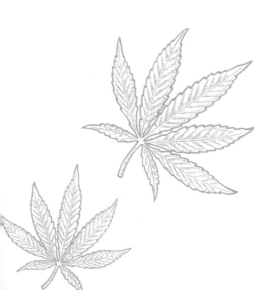

RECOMMENDED PLANTS FOR TEAS

Most fast-growing tall plants that are thriving in your area make great candidates for plant teas. For a more complete list, look up "dynamic accumulator" plants for additional options. Dynamic accumulator plants gather minerals and nutrients from the soil and store them in their tissues. When these plants are used as teas or mulch, or added to compost, these nutrients and minerals become available for the plants in your garden and can be absorbed more easily.

Alfalfa	Comfrey	Pigweed
Borage	Curly dock	Sage
Burdock	Dandelion	Skullcap
Calendula	Feverfew	Stinging nettle (one of the best plants to use for all stages of growth)
Chickweed	Garlic mustard	
Chicory	Horsetail	
Chives	Male cannabis plants	Yarrow

Compost and Manure Teas

Just as you can use plants to brew a nutritious tea for your plants, you can also make teas using compost and manure. Also known as liquid compost and manure, these mixtures act as a mild, high-nitrogen, microbe-rich fertilizer that can be used throughout the growing season, especially during the vegetative stage. They are easy to brew, and the nutrients from compost and manure readily dissolve in water. Liquid compost and manure can be applied via a watering can or a sprayer. Any excess debris from your tea can then be added back into your compost pile or spread onto the surface of the soil.

A quick internet search will reveal sources of compost or manure in your area. If you live near a rural area, you can ask local farmers if they have any manure for sale. I recommend sourcing manure from animals that have been raised organically and have not been fed growth hormones or antibiotics. If you only need a small amount, you can always purchase some bagged compost or manure from your local garden center.

It is important to use fully decomposed compost or manure. Fresh manure needs to sit in a pile for 8–12 months to decompose and be safe to use. Turning the pile once or twice during this time will help to break it down more quickly. Bagged compost and manure have usually been broken down and are ready to use right away.

Homemade Liquid Compost and Manure

YIELD: 5 gallons (19 L)

What You Need

Compost, manure, or a mixture of both, approximately 2½ gallons (9.5 L) or enough to fill the 5-gallon (19-L) bucket halfway

Water

Air pump or aerator (see page 24)

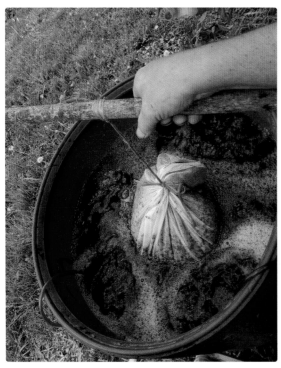

The ingredients of this tea (compost and worm castings) are held in a mesh paint strainer bag, which can be found at home improvement stores. Burlap bags can also be used for this purpose.

1. Fill up a 5-gallon (19-L) bucket halfway with compost, manure, or a mixture of both. You can place the compost and manure in a burlap sack or pillowcase to create a "'tea bag." Fill the remaining half of the bucket with water, making sure to cover all the plant material.

2. Cover with a lid and set the bucket outside. Aerate this mixture with an air pump to help keep it oxygenated. Let this mixture sit with the air pump on for 2–3 days and stir it a handful of times each day. After 2–3 days, it will be ready to use. The water will have changed to a dark brown color. (This exact color may vary, depending on the type of compost or manure you used.) There may be some bubbles that have formed on the surface.

3. When the tea is ready, let the solids sink to the bottom or pull out your tea bag and squeeze out all that liquid goodness.

4. To use when watering, dilute this tea at a ratio of 1 part tea to 10 parts water. To use as a foliar spray, create a mixture at a ratio of 1 part tea to 40 parts water and pour it into a spray bottle. (The mixture should look light brown after it has been diluted.) The diluted solution can be used once every 7–10 days during vegetative growth. It can also be mixed with fermented plant tea (see recipe on page 133).

STORAGE: This tea should be used within 1–2 days after it has been brewed. If you wish to store it for a couple of extra days, make sure that you use an air pump to oxygenate the liquid.

Fish Fertilizer

Fish fertilizer helps to increase soil health and fertility. It is high in nitrogen, it contains phosphorus and potassium, and it should not burn your plants if you apply too much. One of the drawbacks of this product is that it can be smelly, although some manufacturers have produced products that lack the intense smell. (Be sure to research the ingredients that may have been added to remove the smell before buying any.)

There are two main types of fish fertilizers: emulsions and hydrolysates. Fish emulsions have gone through a heat treatment and are products that have had the oils and meal removed. Hydrolysates contain the oils and meal and are cold-pressed. I recommend choosing your fish fertilizer carefully. Some companies use unwanted parts of fish, such as the bones, scales, guts, and heads, while others may harvest and use whole fish. I prefer to support companies that are using unwanted by-products of the fishing industry. If you happen to live near a large body of water or fish yourself, you can research some great recipes for homemade fish fertilizer online as an alternative. They are quite easy to make and work very well.

Bottled Nutrients

If you need to use bottled nutrients (see page 80), I recommend making sure you purchase an organic fertilizer to maintain the health of your soil, your plants, and the planet. When looking for a fertilizer for the vegetative growth stage, purchase one that is high in nitrogen (the N in the N-P-K ratio). Many of these labels will also have the words *grow* or *veg* (as opposed to *bloom* or *flower*). Bottled nutrients will be more expensive than using soil amendments or homemade fertilizers and plant teas.

IDENTIFYING THE SEX OF YOUR PLANTS

Plants in the vegetative stage will begin to show signs of their sex in as little as 4–6 weeks. It is important for you to learn to tell the difference between male and female plants, as it is the flowers or buds of the female plant that you will harvest and your yields will be better if they are not pollinated. If you do not want your cannabis flowers to produce seeds, be sure to remove the male plants from your garden as soon as possible.

Unless you have purchased feminized seeds, there is a good chance you are going to end up with some male plants. Two of the most common methods for determining the sex of your cannabis plants are to wait for the pre-flowers to develop or to take cuttings from your plants and induce them to flower.

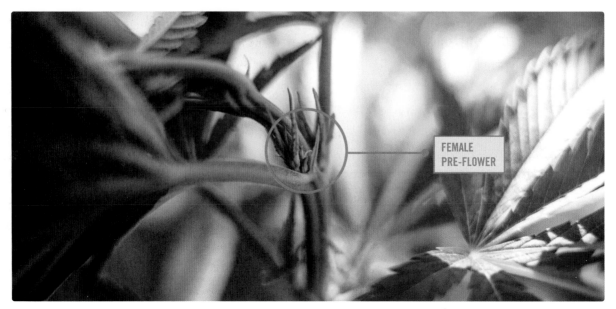

ABOVE This image shows female pre-flowers. You can tell that the plant will be female because there are two pistils forming in the leaf axis. RIGHT This image shows male pre-flowers. Note the circular or "ball-like" structures growing on the leaf axis.

Observing the Pre-flowers

Some plants will begin to show signs of their sex early, at around 4–6 weeks, and some plants will not show any signs as late as 1–2 weeks into the flowering stage. In general, male plants tend to grow faster and taller than females, but this is not a reliable marker of sex. In order to know for sure, you need to examine the pre-flower, which begins to form in the leaf axis (where the leaf stems meet the stalk). It is here that you will first see the hair-like pistils of a female flower or the round ball-like pollen sac of the male flowers. It can be helpful to have a hand lens with ten to thirty times magnification or a jeweler's loupe to look for pre-flowers,

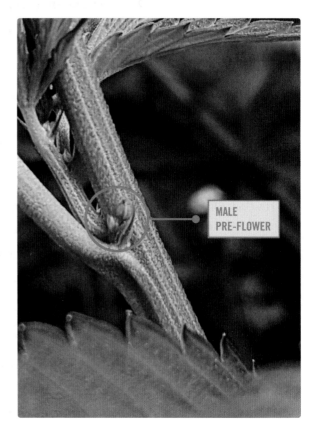

but it is not necessary. Once they have developed further, you should have no problem seeing these signs with the naked eye.

After the first male pre-flower becomes visible, it will take about 10 days to 2 weeks for the male calyx to open and the pollen sacs to appear. Once the sacs appear, the first ones may open within 24 hours. When open, they will drop pollen. For most people, it is important to get rid of the male plants or keep them separated from female plants before this happens.

CULLING HERMAPHRODITE PLANTS

If you see both male and female flowers on the same plant, then it is a hermaphrodite plant. Signs of hermaphroditism generally will not appear until later in the flowering stage, but you may see these signs sooner.

Hermaphrodite plants are very undesirable, and it is best to cull these plants from your garden by cutting them off at the base. You can put them in your compost or make a plant tea (see page 132) with them. The male flowers will pollinate the female flowers of other plants and produce seeds. They will also pass a genetic tendency toward hermaphroditism down to their offspring. You do not want to have these plants pollinate others in your garden and spoil your entire crop.

Cloning for Sex

Another surefire technique for distinguishing male plants from female plants is to take cuttings from each of your plants. Label both the parent plants and the cuttings. Once the cuttings have rooted, you can then induce flowering by giving them 12 hours of light and 12 hours of darkness daily. Within 7–10 days, pre-flowers will begin to form, and you will be able to tell if it is male or female by examining them. You can then either separate your males for breeding or discard the males and focus your energy on the females.

TRAINING AND PRUNING TECHNIQUES TO INCREASE YIELDS

There are a number of pinching, pruning, bending, and training techniques that increase yields by increasing the number of branches or flowering sites at the plant's canopy. Instead of having one main cola (the tallest growing shoot), you can create many "leading" branches. Your plant will become bushier as opposed to having a pyramid-like shape with a single cola.

Some of these techniques are easy to use; the new grower will easily achieve the desired outcomes. Other techniques are better suited for the more experienced grower. I advise you to start with the easier training and pruning techniques and move into some of the more advanced ones after you gain more skill and experience. There

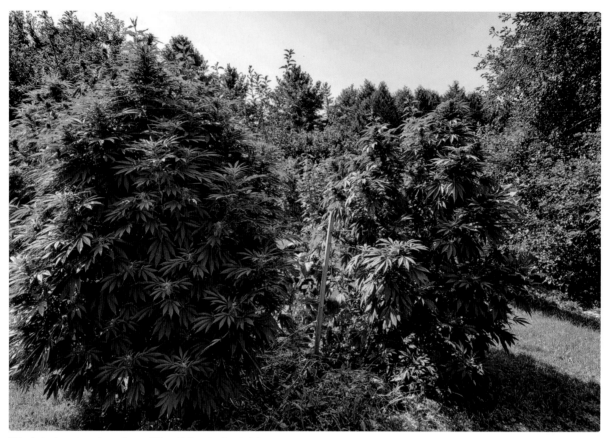

This photo shows two plants that could benefit from having their bottom branches pruned. This allows the cannabis to send more energy to the top of the plant. These plants can also use some defoliating, the process of removing fan leaves to increase airflow and expose flowering sites to sunlight. Both practices can increase your harvest when performed properly.

is an optimum window of time to use some techniques, and sometimes it is possible to use a technique several times throughout the growing season. I will note this in the text below.

I always recommend trying these techniques on one plant at a time and observing the results of your work before carrying out the same procedure on your entire crop. Some cultivars will do better than others with these training techniques. The health of your plant will play a factor as well. Let

your observations guide you, go slowly, and soon these skills will become second nature to you.

Low-Stress Training Techniques

Low-stress training (LST) techniques are a good place for the new grower to increase yields and gain some experience working with cannabis plants. As the name suggests, these methods are not very stressful to the plant and do not suspend their growth for long, if at all.

Bending

One of the simplest techniques for obtaining more flowering sites is to bend your plants so that all the side branches receive more light. This causes them to direct growth hormones between all the side branches. As a result, the branches grow vertically, eventually giving you multiple colas, instead of just one.

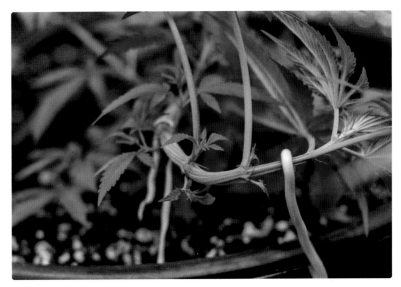

Bending a young cannabis plant allows it to receive more light along its side branches and take on a "bushier" form. This technique can be used with larger plants in the vegetative stage as well.

There are a number of ways that you can bend your plants. You can use twine, plant ties, or rubber-coated wire to tie a loop around the stem of your plant and the other end of the twine, tie, or wire to a pot. You can also weigh the end down or use landscape staples, tent pegs, or a stick to anchor the string when growing in the ground. Alternatively, you can put a bamboo or wooden stake into the ground at a 45-degree angle, slowly bend the plant down toward the stake, and then tie it off. When using these methods, always be careful not to tie your strings or wire too tightly around the stem of the plant, as this could choke off the flow of water and nutrients, ultimately killing the branch or even the entire plant.

After about 10 days, your plant will be trained to grow in this manner, and you can untie it. The plant's stem will continue to grow much bigger during the season and can quickly fill up the space around the string or plant tie that you tied around the stem. Because of this, I recommend that you take these strings or wires off your plants once they have been trained.

The best time for bending your plants is when they are young, as they will be a lot more flexible. You can always try this when they are older as well, but it is very easy to snap and break branches of older plants. Some partially broken branches will heal themselves with some help. To accelerate the healing process, you can use zip ties or string to hold the broken limb in the position it was in before the break. Sometimes using a piece of bamboo as a splint can be helpful. If the break is not too severe, the plant should heal itself in about 7–10 days. If the broken branch dies, you will need to cut it off and discard it in the compost pile.

Leaf Tucking

Another simple LST method is to tuck large leaves underneath other leaves to expose more flower sites to light. Once you tuck or fold the leaves, they should stay where they are; there is no need to tie them off. If you choose to use this technique, you will have to continue doing so as the plant grows.

It is fine to simply break or pinch off some of the fan leaves during the vegetative cycle to expose flowering sites to light. Just be sure to only take a few off at a time if your plants are under 2 feet (61 cm) tall. When removing leaves, break them off cleanly at the point where the leaf is attached to the stem, being sure not to leave part of the petiole sticking out from the stem. These short pieces can increase the likelihood that diseases such as botrytis (see page 215) will take hold.

Screen of Green

The screen of green (ScrOG) method uses trellis netting suspended horizontally over your plants. Your plants will grow into the netting, and you can bend them down and back under the netting to allow more flower sites to receive light.

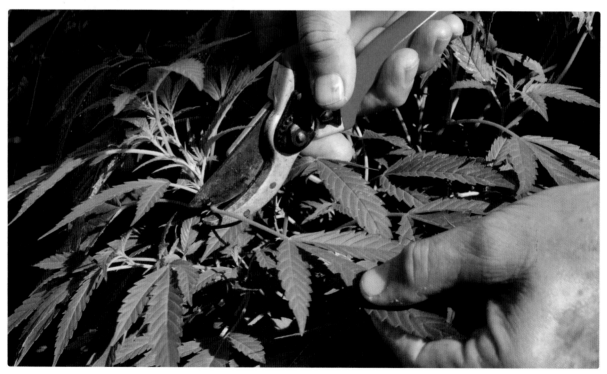

If you want to remove fan leaves, you can use a hand pruner (*as shown here*), scissors, or your hands. Be sure to make a clean cut and break off the leaf as close to the main stem as possible.

Incorporating this method can greatly increase your yields, while also lending some stability and support for your heavy, bud-ridden plants.

High-Stress Training

High-stress training (HST) often involves breaking or removing parts of your plant. While these methods will initially stall or stunt growth, they can greatly increase yields. These techniques are considered more advanced, and the grower should take great care when using them to ensure that the plants return to normal growth soon after the techniques are applied.

Because HST techniques are hard on your plants, you need to give them some time to recover in between each application. You can continue to employ these techniques throughout the vegetative stage as long as your plants heal and continue to grow.

With high-stress training techniques, always use sharp, clean, and sterilized instruments, and sanitize your tools with rubbing alcohol in between each use. If you have both outdoor and indoor plants, use one set of tools inside and another set outside.

Pinching

Pinching is a common technique utilized by gardeners and horticulturalists the world over. Pinching off a growing tip creates two growing shoots and leads to more flowering sites. It also slows down vertical growth and encourages horizontal growth. This may come in handy if you have limited space, which is often the case for indoor growers, or if you do not want very tall plants.

Because pinching stunts growth, do not use this technique before your plant has at least four nodes or sets of branches, and make sure to only pinch your plants during the vegetative growth stage, not during flowering. If you begin pinching too soon, it will take a long time for the plant to recover, or it might not recover at all. It is best to stop pinching your plant at least 2 weeks before the onset of the flowering stage.

It will take some time, from a few days to a week or more, before the plant rebounds and starts to grow vigorously again. Some plants will respond better than others to this technique, and some plants may do just fine without any kind of pinching at all—it will depend on the genetics of the plant.

You will not do any long-term damage or harm to your plants by pinching them, as long as you do it correctly. If you are unsure about how your plants will respond, and are growing more than one of the same cultivar, I would recommend pinching one of them and not pinching the other. This way you can compare the results of using and forgoing this technique. Some growers will pinch all their plants, and others will leave them to grow naturally. The choice is yours, and you will produce beautiful plants with or without pinching.

Pinching Step-by-Step

What You Need

Cutting tool, such as a razor, a craft knife,
 a scalpel, or scissors
Rubbing alcohol
Cotton balls, cloth, or paper towel

1. Sterilize your cutting tool. Put a little alcohol on a cotton ball, cloth, or paper towel, and rub it over the cutting tool to clean it. Make sure to pay close attention to the blades. Though the technique is called "pinching" because many growers do it with their fingers, I recommend using a sharp blade or scissors the first few times you do this.

2. Identify the place on the plant that you are going to pinch. Then make a clean cut with your tool of choice, being careful to cut the stem of the plant and not to damage the two new growth shoots located at the base of the stem in the leaf axis (see the photo below). The two growth shoots left behind on the plant will now grow into two shoots and eventually turn into branches. Put the cut branches in your compost pile. You can also dry them out and use them the same way you would use the flower, though they will have a very mild effect.

3. You can choose to continue to pinch your plant as it grows, which will give it more of a bushlike appearance, or you can leave it to grow naturally on its own.

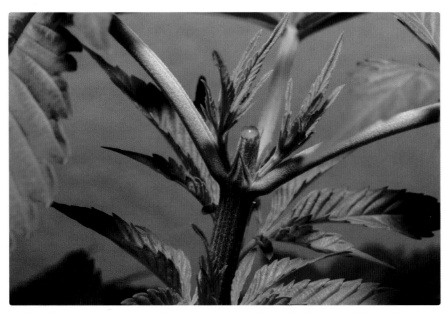

Pinching the tops of a cannabis plant will encourage more branching and lead to a plant with a bushier appearance. Be careful to make as clean a cut as possible.

Fimming

FIM is an acronym that stands for "Fuck, I missed." The term was coined by a grower from South Carolina after he missed the proper spot for pinching his plant. This technique is very similar to the pinching process outlined above, but you cut your plant at a different spot. Whereas pinching takes off the main growing shoot, fimming takes off the upper two-thirds of the growing shoot, leaving one-third on the bottom.

From this cut area, two to four branches will form. The lower branches will grow upward because the cut will redistribute auxin, the plant's growth hormone, to the lower part of the plant, causing the lower branches to grow upward. Your plants should recover in about 2–4 days, and you will see new leaves and growth.

This method of pruning gives your plants a sloppy and careless appearance and does not always produce the desired results. You are also putting your plant at a greater risk of infection because you are not making a clean cut on the stem of the plant, as you do when you are pinching. However, because this technique can result in two extra branches (four in total) as opposed to two branches that are produced when using the pinching technique, some growers will try fimming their plants for this payoff.

RIGHT In this diagram, the orange line indicates where you should cut the growing shoot if you are fimming it, while the blue line indicates how much of the growing shoot you should remove for pinching.

Fimming Step-by-Step

What You Need

Cutting tool, such as a razor, a craft knife,
    a scalpel, or scissors
Rubbing alcohol
Cotton balls, cloth, or paper towel

1. Sterilize your cutting tool. Put a little alcohol on a cotton ball, cloth, or paper towel, and rub it over the cutting tool to clean it. Make sure to pay close attention to the blades.

2. Identify the spot that you wish to cut. Instead of making a cut on the stem, make your cut about two-thirds of the way down the leaves and growing shoots. You will leave the bottom third on the stem.

3. You can choose to continue to fim your plant as it grows, which will give it more of a bushlike appearance, or you can leave it to grow naturally on its own.

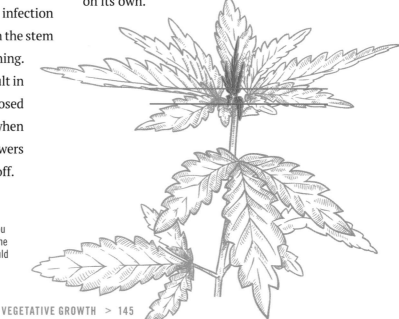

Lollipopping

Lollipopping involves removing the lower branches of the plant. Because they are at the bottom of the plant, these branches do not get enough light to develop large flowers. By pruning them off the plant, the plant will direct more energy to the top branches that are closer to light and produce denser and larger flowers. Lollipopping allows more air to flow through your plants, making them less susceptible to diseases, such as mold and powdery mildew (see page 213). It also allows you to see what is happening with your plant at ground level. As with pruning and fimming, it is important to make a nice, clean cut and not to leave a stump when cutting off branches. Stumps could leave your plant more susceptible to pests or diseases.

You can also just focus on removing the dead, yellow, and discolored leaves. (These leaves may be signs of a nutrient imbalance—see chapter 13). If you grab the leaf with your hand and bend it down toward the ground, it will snap off with a clean break at the base of the stem. In addition to pruning yellow and discolored leaves, you can then remove some of the leaves that are covering flowering sites and branch tips. It is important to find a balance when pruning leaves. Do not take off too many of the fan leaves, as they are needed for photosynthesis, but make sure that there aren't many leaves that prevent light from penetrating the canopy and reaching as many flowering sites as possible.

TIP: When pruning (or any time you work with your plants), it is a good idea to get in the habit of closely observing all your plants. Look for any signs of disease or pests. If they're healthy, celebrate their health and get to know the unique characteristics of every plant. If they are unhealthy, take note of what is happening and create a plan to bring them back to health.

Super Cropping

Super cropping is thought to increase the number of flowering sites, resin production, potency, and yields by prompting the plant's natural stress response. This can be done on multiple branches of the same plant and on both indoor and outdoor plants. Growers roll and squish the stem of the plant between their index finger and thumb, breaking the fibers and causing it to fall over. The plant then grows a hard callus at the site of the injury. This is an advanced technique, as it can damage your plants and potentially make them susceptible to disease.

Super cropping is best done about 1–2 weeks before the flowering stage. More experienced growers can use this technique several times during the vegetative cycle. If you break a stem or do more damage than you wanted to, you can always tie your plant off to a stake or another branch, or use tape and small wooden splints to bandage up the break. It should heal within 7–10 days, at which time you can take the bandage off.

Main-lining

Main-lining, also known as manifolding, is used mostly by indoor growers who want to make the most of a small space. It involves splitting the main growing shoot of the plant to create a Y-shaped branch called a manifold.

To use this technique, you first pinch your plant to create two growing shoots. You then tie or weigh down each of those growing shoots, creating a Y-shaped split. You can continue to pinch and tie down the growing shoots as many times as you want, but most people will stop after about 3 weeks and transition their plants into the flowering stage. This technique will increase the number of branches and flowers, ultimately leading to higher yields. It also creates better airflow through your plant and allows each flower site to receive the optimal amount of light.

PROVIDING SUPPORT

During the vegetative stage, you will want to offer extra support for your plants as they grow and prepare for flowering. The more support the branches have, the more energy they will put into making the biggest, most dense flowers. The form of support can be as simple as sticking a wooden stake or a piece or bamboo into the ground and tying the stem to it, or it could mean assembling cages. In some cases, you may want to trellis your plant.

Fully mature cannabis flowers are very top-heavy and weigh more than you may think, especially when wet. Without additional support, some large plants can easily topple over and break off at the main stem during a windstorm. You do not want this to happen to even one plant—let alone an entire crop. Depending on the genetics of your plants, their size, and your local weather, you may not need to stake or trellis them. But it is better to be safe than sorry, especially with your first crop. An ounce of prevention is worth a pound of cure. Support your plants—it is a very important step that you do not want to skip!

Wooden Stakes and Bamboo

Putting a wooden stake or a piece of bamboo beside your plant and then tying the plant to the stake is a great way to secure your plants. This can be especially helpful in windy locations. As your plant grows, you may need to tie it off again near the top of the plant or attach an extension to the stake.

Wire Cages

Many people put a wire cage around their plants and then let the plants grow through the fencing. The fencing acts as a trellis, offering support to the branches. You can also manipulate and spread out your branches by encouraging them to grow through specific sections of the fencing.

As your plants grow, you may wish to add another layer of fencing outside the original one. You can even use another piece of fencing to extend the height of your cage, if your plants are really taking off.

Trellis Netting and Rope

Trellising involves installing netting, often made from jute or plastic. The netting is stretched over the canopy of your plants. The branches of your plants will grow through the netting, and the netting will stabilize and support them, especially after flowers form.

You may choose to place a layer of trellis netting horizontally across the canopy of your plants. You can set up the netting by arranging four or six stakes around your plants, pulling the netting tightly over the plants, and securing it to the stakes. Some growers will add two or even three layers of trellis netting as the plant grows toward the sun, since multiple layers of netting can provide more support for larger plants. As with wire cages, you can pull the branches apart and direct them through various holes in the netting to train them to grow a certain way.

High-Tensile Wire

Depending on how you plant your cannabis, you can also use high-tensile wire to support your plants and keep them from blowing over in wind- and rainstorms. You will need to string wire between two or more anchor points that run downwind of the prevailing winds in your area, either alongside or through the center of your plants. Alternatively, you could also run two wires, one down each side of your plants, giving them support from two sides.

This technique works best when growing plants in rows, and it can be done so the wire is hardly noticeable to the human eye.

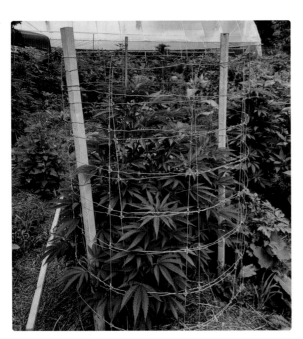
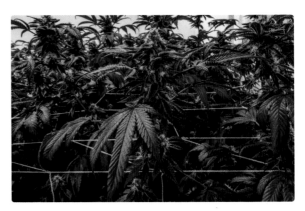

A wire cage (*left photo*) provides support by offering something for the branches of your plants to lean on. It also supports the main stem of the plant. Trellis netting (*right photo*) is often placed horizontally across cannabis to provide growing plants, which will become top-heavy when they flower, with extra support.

FAQS & TROUBLESHOOTING

Q: Why are my plants growing slowly?

A: Your plants need adequate amounts of sunlight, carbon dioxide, nutrients, and water to maintain optimal growth. Slow growth often results from deficiencies in one or more of these factors. Here are some possible explanations:

- Your plants are not getting enough light.
- Your plants may need more nutrients or fertilizer.
- The temperature may be too hot or too cold.
- Your plants may be over- or underwatered.
- Your plants are stressed or stunted. If this happens, it can take a week or more for normal growth to resume.
- If they are in pots, your plants could be root-bound and need to be transplanted into a larger pot.
- Some plants are runts, or they could just be slow-growing plants.

Q: Can I just let my plants grow naturally and skip training?

A: Yes. You should try it and see what happens. All the techniques featured in this chapter are just that—techniques. They do not have to be used to grow great cannabis. Sometimes it is best to simply let your plant grow au naturel. I recommend leaving a plant or two to grow on its own and then employ one or two of the techniques mentioned in this chapter with the other plants. This way, you can compare and contrast the results and gain experience with a number of different techniques over the course of one growing season.

Q: Why are the leaves of my plants turning yellow? Is something wrong?

A: There could be many reasons that the leaves of your plants are turning yellow. Some of the most common include nitrogen deficiency (see page 219), over- or underwatering, or your plant becoming root-bound. Also be on the lookout for any pests that may be damaging your plant.

Q: How can I protect my outdoor plants if there is severe weather, such as a heat wave or a severe windstorm?

A: There are a number of environmental factors that can cause stress to your plants. In terms of heat waves and intense sunlight, you may be able to shade your plants (see page 103 to learn how). If your plants are large and healthy, they should be able to withstand heat waves and intense sunlight as long as you keep them watered and they do not dry out. Windstorms are common in some areas, and the best way to protect against this is to make sure your plants are supported well with bamboo and wooden stakes and cages. The better supported they are, the less likely they will be to break, bend, or fall over. Making sure that your plants have all the nutrients they need in the soil will also allow them to be strong and resilient in the face of any inclement weather or adverse environmental conditions.

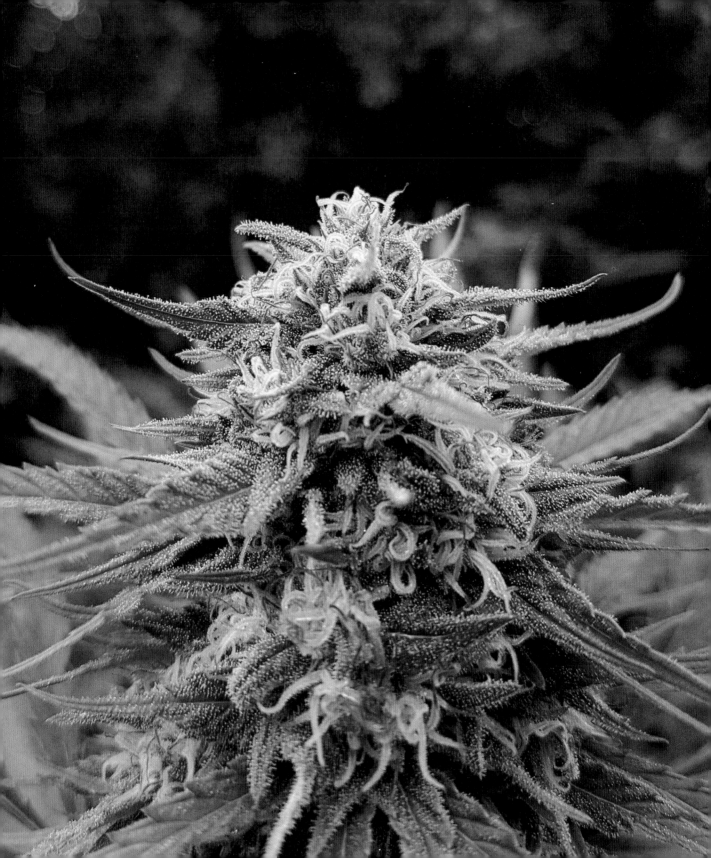

CHAPTER 9

< Flowering >

The flowering stage is one of the most exciting times for the cannabis grower. In this stage, your plants experience some of the most dramatic changes in the growing season. It is a time of transformation, beauty, and the unveiling of a plant's potential. No matter how many years or plants a person has grown, every grower gets excited as their plants leave the vegetative stage and enter the flowering stage.

SIGNS OF FLOWERING

Before your cannabis begins to flower, your plant will enter what some people refer to as the "early flower stretch." During these first couple of weeks of the flowering cycle, your plants will begin to experience quick and robust growth in the stems and branches in anticipation of the heavy flowers to come.

The flowers or buds will then begin to appear, starting at the tip of the branches and then moving down and filling out the rest of the plant. You will get to see the color and form of the pistils. They can be white, red, or many other colors. They can be long or short, dense, or spaced out. The buds will get bigger and bigger each day as you approach harvest, and the shape, size, and density of the flowers will increase as they put on both mass and weight. Colas will emerge. Some plants can produce dozens, even hundreds of these prized colas!

Trichomes will form in dense arrangements all over the flowers and leaves. Terpenes, found in the plant's trichomes, give cannabis its many unique smells, and many a grower cannot walk by this special plant without taking a big inhale of the beautiful scents that emanate from its

LEFT This Afghan Hash Plant is in full flower, but it is still a couple weeks away from harvest. The small white bumps on the buds are trichomes.

< 151 >

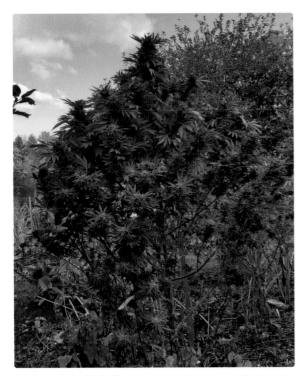

This Lemon Cake x Trinity Kush plant is about a week away from harvest. The orange tag marks a bottom branch with pollinated flowers that will produce seeds for next year.

precious flowers. Each cultivar has a distinctive smell that can include lemon, gas, skunk, fruit, floral, piney, spicy, and earthy flavors.

You may find that once the buds start to form, your plants will grow rapidly for the next 4–5 weeks, swelling and putting on mass. They will then slow in growth, and over the next 2–3 weeks of flowering, your plants will get denser, put on a lot of weight, and fully fill out. Healthy plants can almost double the weight of their buds in these last few weeks, so it is important to give them this time to mature whenever possible. Trust me, it will be more than worth it, though sometimes,

bad weather will force you to harvest earlier than you would like.

Different cultivars flower at different times. Some seed companies may state on the package or in the description on their website the number of days or weeks each cultivar will take to flower. If you get your seeds or clones from other growers, they may have this information to share with you as well. The majority of outdoor cannabis flowers in time for harvesting between October and mid-November. (October is often referred to as "Croptober.") Many of the BLD varieties have evolved to flower earlier and may be ready to harvest outdoors in early to mid-September. On the other hand, some of the NLD varieties may not be ready until late November, even into December. There are also many hybrid varieties that are ready to harvest between those months.

Although you will be able to determine the sex for most plants by their pre-flowers (see page 137), some male plants may hold out on revealing their sex until the flowering stage. This is one reason you should always monitor the plants that have not been identified as females. Don't assume that your plants are female until you have observed pistils and small buds forming.

TIP: Observe and record in your plant journal how much your plants grow as they approach flowering, when they begin flowering, and when they are ready for harvest. This information will be invaluable in subsequent years.

PLANT CARE FOR FLOWERING

As your plants begin to enter the flowering stage, it is important to make sure they have all the nutrients they need to fully mature and reach their peak potential. You also want to make sure you keep a close eye on all your plants: Take note of how they are growing, and make sure they are not becoming susceptible to disease, pests, or lack of airflow. It is important to make sure that your plants have everything they need to fully develop, even if you cannot control the weather.

Lighting

Indoor growers can induce flowering any time by changing the light cycle to 12 hours of light and 12 hours of darkness. If you're growing plants outside, the latitude at which you live will affect flowering. As summer turns to fall, the amount of daylight decreases. The farther north you go in the summer, the longer the days are, resulting in more daylight available for plants. As a result, plants grown in northern climates will begin flowering later than plants grown farther south, even if they are the same cultivar.

In most locations, cannabis will start to flower between late July and late August. I live at approximately 44°6'58" in Great Lakes country in southern Ontario. Our plants generally start to flower around August 5–15, with some cultivars starting a little before or after this time frame. Those of us here in the north try to harvest our cannabis

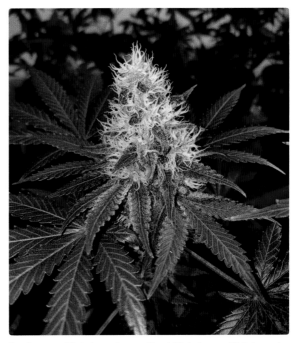

Growing cannabis indoors gives you the ability to have multiple harvests throughout the year and to transition your plants into the flowering stage whenever you want.

around the first week of October. Sometimes we can push the harvest to mid-October or beyond, but the weather can get dicey at this time of year, and there may be frost as well as many days of cool, wet weather.

Although you may not be able to change the weather and conditions in your geographic location, you can choose the cultivars that you grow and match them to your regional conditions. As time goes by, pay attention to how your plants do in your area, especially if you grow cannabis for several seasons. In a few short years, you will have a very good idea of which plants will thrive in your specific zone.

Growing Conditions

For indoor plants, the temperature of your grow space should stay consistently around 72°F–76°F (22°C–24°C). You can allow the nights to get cooler near the end of flowering stage with temperatures of 65–70°F (18–21°C). Allowing this to happen just before harvest will mimic what happens naturally outside during fall. For some cultivars, these conditions may bring out the purple hues of the leaves and flowers and potentially increase yield and potency. The humidity should fall between 40 and 50 percent. It is important to monitor humidity to avoid excess moisture in your room, which will prevent mold.

When growing outdoors, it is important to keep an eye on the weather forecast, especially so you can plan your harvesting accordingly. In most cases, outdoor plants are a lot more resilient when it comes to temperature and humidity swings than indoor plants. Many cultivars can withstand cold temperatures and even a light frost or two, but you do not want to combine cold and frost with prolonged periods of wet weather. It is best to harvest your plants a little early than run the risk of losing them to a "killing" frost.

Watering

Your plants will not typically need as much water during this stage, so be careful not to overwater. For outdoor plants, I recommend skipping watering for the last 10 days of the flowering period, unless they show signs of dehydration, such as drooping leaves. If your plants are in pots or indoors, let them dry out almost completely in between waterings for the same period and try to avoid watering at all in the few days just before harvesting. Don't worry if it rains during this time or you end up needing to give your plants water—they will still do just fine.

Nutrition

As your plants move from the vegetative to flowering stage, they will need less nitrogen and more phosphorus, potassium, and calcium. If you are not working with living soil or just want to give your plants a boost, you can help deliver these nutrients to the plants at this time.

Your plants will let you know if they are missing something. If your flowers are growing exceedingly slowly or are not putting on a large amount of mass, they could be in need of more phosphorus and potassium. If the branches are weak and break easily, the petioles turn red, and reddish-brown spots develop on your leaves, they might be in need of more calcium and magnesium.

Just before flowering really takes off, it is important for your plants to have enough nitrogen, phosphorus, and calcium so that they can increase stem and branch strength and develop numerous bud sites. You may choose to top-dress your soil with compost or deliver these nutrients to your plants via manure teas, if they are not already incorporated into your soil mix, or water-soluble calcium (see page 155).

Water-Soluble Calcium

This gentle solution of water-soluble calcium (WSC) offers a highly bioavailable source of this important nutrient to your plants. It can be used for watering or as a foliar spray. You can use WSC as the plant transitions to flowering and throughout the flowering stage. If you're using it for the transition phase, you can pair the water-soluble calcium with manure teas, especially those made with chicken manure, but stop adding the manure teas once flowering has begun.

YIELD: About 4¼ cups (1 L)

What You Need

1 cup eggshells, cleaned, dried, and crushed

2 (½-gallon [2-L]) glass jars, with lids

4¼ cups (1 L) rice vinegar or apple cider vinegar

Paper towels, a dish towel, or cheesecloth

Funnel and strainer

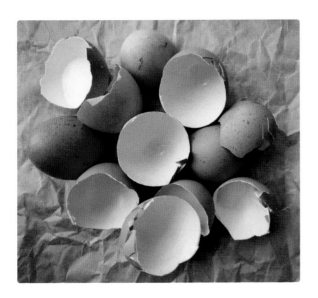

Note: You can make a water-soluble calcium phosphate solution by using animal bones instead of eggshells. Clean the bones of any skin, flesh, or fat by boiling them for a few hours. (You can also leave them outside and let the weather and various insects clean them for you.) Char the bones in a fire and then crush the charred bones into smaller pieces. From here, follow steps 3–5.

1. In a pan placed on an outdoor grill, cook the eggshells over high heat. (You can cook them inside, but it will be a little smelly without an overhead fan.) Cover the pan and let them cook for approximately 45 minutes to 1 hour, until they are brown and extremely brittle, stirring them several times as they cook.

2. As the eggshells cook, you can remove the membrane on the underside of the eggshells by fanning them as they cook and letting the membranes "fly" out. This is easiest if you are cooking them outside. Once the eggshells are brown and thoroughly cooked, remove them from the heat and let them cool. You can also remove the membrane after the eggshells have cooked and once they have cooled down. Transfer them to another bowl and swish the eggshells around while gently blowing on the membranes so they fly off.

3. Place the eggshells in one glass container and slowly pour the vinegar into the same container. The mixture will foam and produce bubbles, so be careful not to pour too quickly. Cover the container with paper

towels, a dish towel, or cheesecloth, and secure it with an elastic band. Label the container with the date.

4. Leave the mixture for 5–7 days (up to 10 days is fine), at room temperature and out of direct sunlight. The eggshells will rise and fall for the first few days as a result of a chemical reaction between the calcium and the vinegar. If there is no reaction, this means that you have not cooked the eggshells long enough, and you will have to start over.

5. With a funnel and a strainer, pour the liquid into a clean container. Put a lid on the container and label it. Add the leftover eggshells to your garden soil, compost, or worm bin. Like the LABS serum, WSC needs to be diluted at a ratio of 1:1000 before using as a foliar spray. See the dilution ratio chart on page 70. You can use it at about twice the strength for watering directly into the soil using a ratio of 1:500, two or three times over the course of the flowering stage. If you're using it as a foliar spray, apply once every 5–7 days during the first 2–3 weeks of flowering when the flowers are just starting to form.

STORAGE: This solution is shelf-stable and will last for at least a year. If you used a living or homemade vinegar, leave the cap cracked a bit.

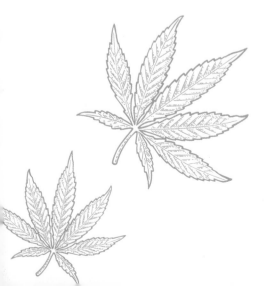

When buds are forming, your plants are going to need more phosphorus, potassium, and calcium. At this time, you can continue to feed them the water-soluble calcium and liquid bone meal (both of which provide calcium and phosphate). If you're using fermented plant teas (see recipe on page 133), consider brewing them with plants high in phosphorus and potassium, such as mugwort (*Artemesia vulgaris*), lambsquarters (*Chenopodium album*), pigweeds (*Amaranthus* spp.), feverfew (*Chrysanthemum parthenium*), dandelion (*Taraxacum officinale*), chicory (*Cichorium intybus*), horsetail (*Equisetum arvense*), stinging nettle (*Urtica dioica*), sumac (*Rhus* spp.), and wild grape (*Vitis* spp.).

In the final stage of flowering, make sure your plants get ample amounts of potassium, calcium, and carbohydrates. It is also a good idea to water with a fermented plant tea made from aromatic herbs, such as chamomile, rosemary, oregano, tulsi, lemon balm, thyme, and calendula. You can add many of the flowering plants from your local area or gardens into your plant teas as well. Sunflowers, zinnias, old cannabis flowers, and a plethora of other plants in flower at this time of year make great additions.

Following this feeding regimen will give your flowers an amazing smell and taste. During the last 7–10 days of flowering, I do not recommend giving your plants anything except water and only water if you have to. They will produce more resin and trichomes if they experience a little drought stress right at the end of flowering.

Maintenance

During flowering, you can continue to prune leaves that have become diseased or discolored, or have died back. You can also remove leaves covering flowering sites or very densely arranged, but make sure not to take off too many. These discarded leaves are best left on top of your soil (near the base of your plant), to let the nutrients and minerals within them go back into the earth.

As your flowers increase in size, make sure that you have supported your plants with cages or stakes earlier in the vegetative stage. You do not want them to fall or blow over under the increased weight of their flowers. It is a shame to see branches full of immature flowers fall and break from the plant. See pages 147–148 for some recommended methods.

THE BASICS OF BREEDING

Although breeding cannabis (and any plant for that matter) is a topic that could take up an entire book, I would like to give you a brief primer in case you have the time and space to grow a few extra plants for this purpose. Producing seeds is one of the most rewarding and regenerative practices you can do as a grower. It is a skill that is being forgotten by far too many people and one that offers self-reliance.

Be aware that the quality of your flowers will suffer if they are pollinated as the plant will put its energy into producing seeds as opposed to flowers. You will still be able to use your flowers, but they will not be as potent or taste as good. I recommend that you choose flowers from one branch to hand-pollinate and leave the rest of the plant to ripen without seeds.

Choosing Parent Plants

Breeding can be as simple as "chucking" some pollen from a male plant onto a female plant. (A "pollen chucker" is a person who haphazardly spreads pollen around a garden.) However, it is best to give some intentional thought to your breeding plans. There are many factors that you may want to consider when picking two plants to breed with. Here are a few:

- **Phenotype:** Think about the phenotype you want your new plant to display. A phenotype is the set of traits that your plant displays. For example, you may prefer the plant to grow to a specific height, exhibit a particular branching pattern, or have a smell or color that you like. Many cannabis growers will conduct "pheno" hunts, which involves looking through a large number of plants for desirable traits. When you're ready to choose plants for breeding, look for male and female plants with these traits, though you may observe certain traits only in the male or female plant. You can cross two plants with traits similar to the

ones that you want, or cross a plant with a certain characteristic with one of its parents in hopes that the trait will show up in the next generation.

- **Potency:** You may want to increase the THC or CBD content in the next generation of plants. This would involve crossing a high-potency cultivar with another one of lesser potency.

- **Pest- and disease-resistance:** Whether because of their chemical makeup or genetics, some plants will have built-in resistance to common pests or diseases, making them good candidates for a breeding project. For example, many breeders will breed for plants that are resistant to powdery mildew, botrytis, spider mites, or aphids.

- **Finishing times:** Depending where you live, you may want to create plants that finish earlier or later in the season.

- **Creating a new cultivar:** You may choose to create a new cultivar or continue the filial generation of the cultivar that you are working with. Crossing two unique cultivars will make a new F1 hybrid. An F1 hybrid is the first filial generation that results from breeding two different parent plants. An F2 is made when you breed the F1 hybrid with another F1 from the same generation of seeds.

Pollination Methods

You will need to have at least one male plant in your garden or at least the pollen from one to pollinate your female flowers. There are a couple of options for pollination to consider when you are planning your breeding project.

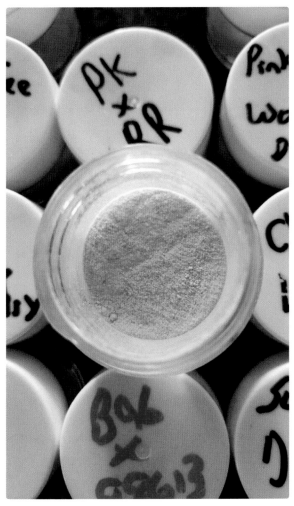

Once collected and dried, store pollen in jars labeled with the collection date and the name of the cultivar from which you took the pollen. The pollen in the open container came from a few branches of a male plant.

Open pollination breeding: For this easy and straightforward option, plant one or more male plants in the same area as one or more female plants. Your female plants should be downwind from the male plants, approximately 3–15 feet (1–4.5 m) apart or more if you are pollinating a lot of plants. The pollination of the female plants will happen naturally as the male releases pollen. You will not want all your female plants in the same vicinity if you do not want each one to produce seeds. Pollen can travel great distances on the wind!

Hand pollination: This method involves growing a male plant away from your female plants. Once most of the flowers are about to open, you will gather the pollen. Cut 12- to 16-inch (30- to 40-cm) long branches off the plant, trim off the fan leaves, and place them in a vase with water indoors. Place the vase on top of a piece of parchment paper and simply allow the pollen to fall onto the paper. (You can angle the jar and gently tap the flower stalks to encourage the pollen to fall as well.) Allow this pollen to dry for a couple of days, then scrape it off the paper and strain it through a kitchen sieve or screen to remove any flower parts, which can lead to spoilage. Another option is to place branches into a paper or plastic bag and vigorously shake the branch to deposit the pollen into the bag. You can do this while the plant is in the ground; just be sure to let the pollen dry before straining it and sealing it in the bag or another container. After you have collected this pollen, it can be used right away or stored in a jar with a tight-fitting lid. It will keep in the fridge for about a month or in the freezer for up to a year.

When you are ready to pollinate, dip a small paintbrush into the pollen and then rub it onto the pistils of the female flowers. This method allows you to pollinate just one or two branches on your female plants so that you can harvest and use the other flowers growing on the plant. Be sure to mark the branches that you pollinated with a piece of flagging tape and note the name of the plant where the pollen came from.

Once the female plant has received pollen, the pistils should begin to die back and change to an orange or brown color. This signifies that the pollen has traveled down the pistil, and the seed formation will begin in the ovary, which is located inside the calyx. The calyx forms a little "pod" that houses the seed as it develops. As the seed grows, the "pod" will expand and grow with it.

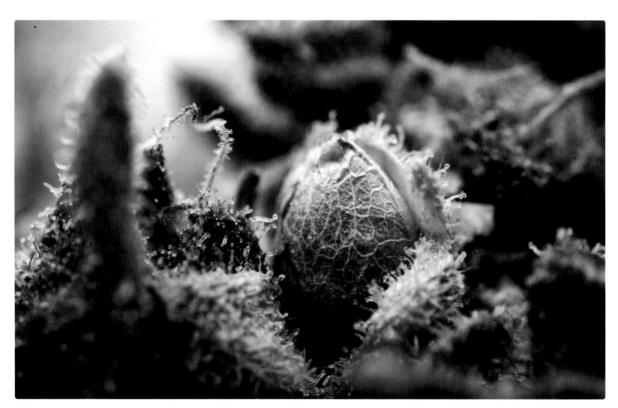

It is best to leave cannabis seeds on the live plant until they are mature. Otherwise, you run the risk of collecting immature seeds that will not sprout.

It generally takes 4–6 weeks to produce a viable seed. Viable, mature seeds should be brown in color; most will have black stripes. Immature seeds will be pale or white and will most often feel light and hollow compared to mature seeds. It is best to leave your seeded plants in the ground as long as you can to make sure they have enough time to mature.

TIP: If you're not sure whether your seeds are mature, simply pick off a few seeds. Squish them using your index finger and thumb to remove the seed casing. If they are not brown in color, with dark stripes, they need more time to mature.

Seed Collection and Storage

When you are confident that your seeds are mature, it is now time to harvest the branches with the seeds. I recommend drying the seed branches just as you would your flowers (see chapter 11 for more details on how to do this). The seeds should remain in the flowers without falling out unless your plants were overmature and the branches have begun to die back or show signs of discoloration and even mold. If some seeds are falling out, you can put a blanket or tray below the branches to catch them.

Once the plants are dry, you can store the buds with the seeds in them or break them apart to collect the seeds and store them separately. The buds

can still be used as medicine or even for smoking or vaping, but they will not be top-quality.

If you decide to pull the seeds out of your flowers when they are fresh, you will need to dry the seeds before storing them. You can do this by spreading the seeds out on a screen or a sheet of paper for 10–12 days in an environment that is 45–55 percent humidity and above 64°F (18°C). No matter what method you choose, the seeds need to be dried before storing. If they are sealed up into containers too soon, you run the risk of the seeds developing mold or other pathogens.

It is best to store your dried seeds in a sealed, airtight container in a dark, cool, and dry space that cannot be accessed by insects or small rodents. The most ideal temperature and humidity levels are 43°F–46°F (6°C–8°C) and 20–30 percent, respectively. These conditions allow them to stay dormant and keep them from using up the valuable nutrient reserves that they will need to crack, sprout, and grow into healthy, strong plants. For short-term storage (6 months or less), you can keep your seeds in any dark drawer or cupboard that does not experience temperature and humidity fluctuations. For long-term storage (6 months or more), use the refrigerator. You can also store your seeds in the freezer if you know that you will not be using them for a while; the cooler the temperature, the slower the decline of the health and vitality of your seeds. Be careful not to let them thaw and freeze over and over again, or they will lose some of their vitality. When taking seeds out of the freezer, try to separate the ones that you want to sprout and put the others back into the freezer as quickly as possible.

Lastly, remember to label the storage container. This will help you remember what plant they came from. Be sure to list the name of the cultivar of both parents and the date that they were harvested or packaged. Proper labeling will also help you disturb the containers as little as possible. Avoid opening each container to find out what is inside, as this results in a change in temperature and humidity that can affect the seeds.

If stored properly, your seeds will remain viable for years to come and provide you with a continued source of quality genetics! I know people who have decade-old seeds with good germination rates.

> **TIP:** When storing your seeds, you can include a few silica gel beads or grains of rice in a piece of cotton. These will help absorb any excess moisture in the container.

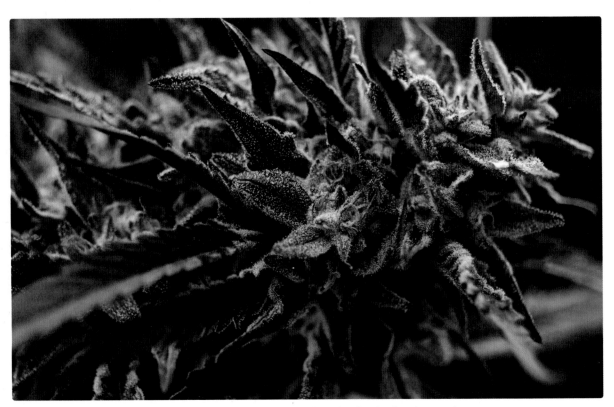

This Mataro Blue x Royal Sour Kush plant was a result of a breeding project and one of my favorite plants in my garden.

FAQS & TROUBLESHOOTING

Q: Why did some of my plants begin flowering early and some not until much later?

A: This mainly has to do with the genetics of the cultivars you chose. Some cultivars have a longer flowering cycle than others and need more time to fully mature, while other plants have shorter flowering cycles and finish early. You always want to look for cultivars that will finish in a time frame that is suitable for your specific growing season conditions. Some growers will grow a few different cultivars to stagger their harvest, while others will choose just one so they can bring in the entire harvest all at once.

Q: How much will my plants smell once they go into flower?

A: The trichome-laden buds can become quite aromatic because of their terpenes. Depending on the cultivar you are growing, they can have a strong odor. Some discerning and aware passersby may be able to detect some strong-smelling plants from 100 feet (30 m) away or more. Most people who use cannabis love the smell that emanates from it, but be aware that this smell can also attract unwelcome and unsavory visitors who may want to steal your precious plants.

Q: My plants started flowering, but the buds seem to be growing slowly and not getting much bigger, and the plant is growing taller. Is this normal?

A: This is fairly common for most cultivars. Once the flowering cycle begins, there is a 10- to 14-day window that is called the "early flowering stretch." A lot of plants will quickly grow taller. Once the flowering stretch is over, the buds will begin to form more quickly. During the last 2 weeks of flowering, you will notice a marked difference as your buds fully mature and put on weight and density. Always let your plants mature as much as possible. By doing so, you will notice greater yield and potency in your final product.

Q: My plants went into the flowering stage in early spring when they were still very small. Why did this happen, and what can I do to keep this from happening again?

A: There are a few things that may have caused this. First, check to see if the seeds you planted were autoflowers, which will flower after a certain period of time has passed. Second, ask yourself if the plants received enough light in the early spring. Some growers try to rely on natural light from a window or greenhouse at this time, but there is not enough daylight in many areas to keep your plant in the vegetative growth stage, especially the farther north you go. In the future, make sure you supply your plants with some supplemental light for a few extra hours each day to prevent them from going into flower when using natural light. Or plant your seeds a little later in the spring season. Some plants may also begin to flower when they are under stress.

If your plants have gone into flower, giving them more light is generally your best option. They will recover, but it may take a couple of weeks or more. Try to remove any sources of stress, and give them the nutrients that they need to be healthy.

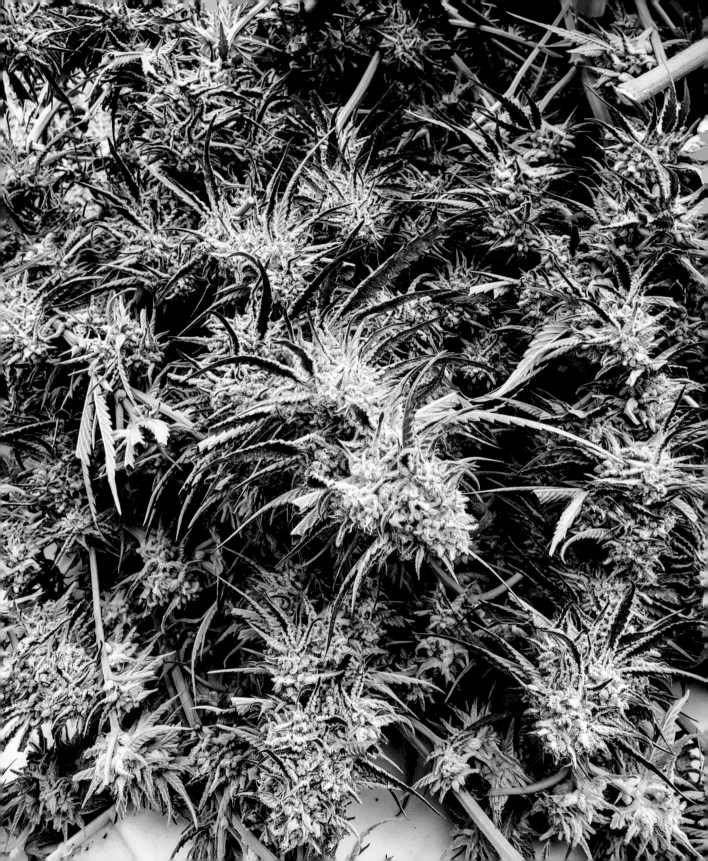

CHAPTER 10

< Harvest >

The harvest is perhaps the most anticipated time of the growing cycle for any cannabis gardener. It is the stage where the plants that you have nurtured, told (select) friends about, and spoke to many times have reached their full maturity. It is a time to celebrate the bounty and beauty of your plants as they reach their full expression. At this point the many hours of tending have paid off, and you will soon be able to enjoy the fruits (or, in this case, the flowers) of your labor. The harvest can also be a time of trepidation, especially for the new gardener who has lots of questions. However daunting and unsure you may be when preparing to harvest your first plants, know that there are many steps that you can take to make sure you can accomplish this task successfully.

WHEN TO HARVEST

As the cannabis plant matures, it begins to focus all its energy on flower production and draws energy away from vertical growth and leaf production so that the flowers can reach their full potential. As this happens, you will notice the following:

- Some leaves may turn yellow (and sometimes purple).

- The pistils change from white to an orange or red. You will harvest when the majority of the pistils have changed color.

- Most of the trichomes have become milky or cloudy in appearance, with some turning amber in color.

LEFT An efficient and stress-free harvest begins with advance planning. It is important to decide how you will transport, store, and dry your buds before cutting down your plants. These flowers came from an Ice Cream Cake x GMO MAC plant.

< 165 >

- The flowers look noticeably denser and heavier and have stopped getting bigger.

- The smell of the flowers is more intense and noticeable at longer distances away from the plants.

Each cultivar is different and can reach maturity at a different time. The most effective way to tell if your plants are ready for harvest is by looking at the trichomes with a hand lens, a jeweler's loupe, or a magnifying glass.

If most of the trichomes are clear, your flowers have not reached their peak potency in terms of their THC or CBD content. If harvested early, the buds will give you a more "cerebral" high that is not felt in the body as much. The color of the trichomes will turn from clear to cloudy or milky when the cannabinoids, such as THC, have reached their peak potency. Amber trichomes are a sign that THC is beginning to degrade. For most plants, the best time to harvest your flowers is when most of the trichomes are cloudy,

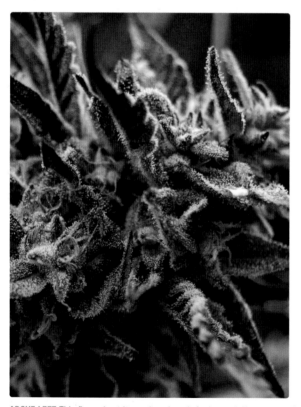 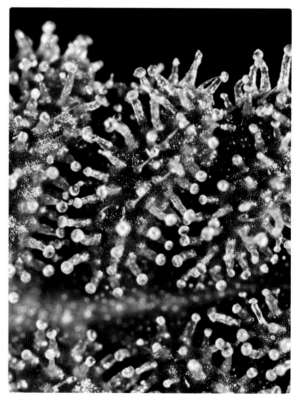

ABOVE LEFT This flower is at its peak and ready for harvest. You can see that the trichomes are cloudy, and there are a few on the leaves that have turned amber. **ABOVE RIGHT** This photo shows how cloudy trichomes will look when viewed with magnification.

and some are beginning to turn amber in color. The flowers will have the highest cannabinoid content at this time. You have about a 7–10-day window to harvest your plants at this peak potency, and it is often the last week or two of the flowering stage when the buds will put on a lot of weight and density.

Once you have determined that your plants are ready to harvest, don't be in a rush and move too quickly. It is best to harvest in the early morning after a few days of hot, sunny weather in order to maximize resin production and to ensure your flowers have the highest levels of cannabinoids and terpenes.

Monitor the trichomes by checking them once a day. If they remain cloudy and are not turning amber too quickly, give the plants some extra time to mature, and your patience will be rewarded with a heavier yield and denser, more compact flowers. It is also a good idea to let your plants dry out as much as possible before harvesting to avoid mold.

HOW TO HARVEST

Being prepared and ready to harvest at the optimal time is very important. Here you will find a detailed look at each of the steps that you need to take to harvest your plants in the best way possible.

HARVESTING AT A GLANCE

1. Make sure you have a plan and know exactly what is going to happen to your plant material once it is harvested.

2. Gather all the tools you will need.

3. Inspect your plants and decide which ones are ready.

4. Prepare your plants for harvesting. If you like, you can de-fan the parts of the plant that you wish to harvest or de-fan when you trim your plants in step 6.

5. Cut down the plants (or the parts of the plants) that you wish to harvest.

6. Trim the big fan leaves (de-fan them). After trimming the fan leaves, your plants are ready for drying. You will also need to decide if you are going to wet- or dry-trim (see page 170 for more details).

Step 1: Make a Plan

Having a well-thought-out plan and preparing a proper drying space in advance can make all the difference between a successful season and an unsuccessful one. The harvest is where many growers go wrong and make mistakes that could have easily been avoided with a solid plan in place. The last thing you want is to cut down your plants and then realize that you do not have anywhere to put them or the right tools or equipment to move on to the next stage of the process. Review the next chapter, where I outline how to set up a proper drying space and discuss many of the parameters for drying your cannabis flowers properly.

Step 2: Gather Your Tools

You'll need handheld pruning shears or loppers, a long-sleeved shirt and pants (as cannabis resin may cause contact dermatitis in some people), tight-fitting gloves, and a bin, tarp, or bag to transport your cannabis from the garden to your drying area. You may also want to have some tape and a marker to label the different cultivars if you have grown more than one kind.

Step 3: Inspect Your Plants

Use the information on pages 165–167 to check if your plants are ready for harvest. The flowers at the tops of your plants will mature faster than the ones at the bottom of your plants. This is simply because the flowers at the top get more energy from the roots and sunlight. Some outdoor gardeners choose to harvest the top portion of their plants and leave the bottom to mature for a few extra days or even weeks. You might do the same, depending on the size of your plants, the weather, the time of year, and the amount of space you have in your drying room.

Step 4: Prepare Your Plants

Many growers, including myself, prefer to de-fan, or remove big leaves before harvesting. You can easily snap these leaves off by clasping the stem of the leaf between your thumb and index finger and simply pulling down toward the ground. Most times, this simple motion will cleanly snap the leaf stem off right at the base.

If you de-fan outside, you don't need to use extra space to dry material that will only be trimmed off later, and you can leave this plant material right in the garden to decompose. If you prefer not to de-fan outside, you can do it after you harvest when you trim the plants just before the drying process (see Step 6: Trim Your Plants, page 170).

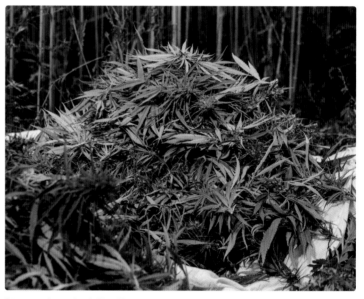

A tarp or a large plastic bin offers a convenient option for transporting your harvest from your garden and into your trimming and drying space.

If you are growing outdoors in living soil, without synthetic nutrients, you do not need to flush your plants before harvesting. Flushing is used mostly by indoor growers who will give their plants excess water a few times before harvesting to remove any buildup of nutrients from the soil and the plant itself. If you are growing indoors in pots, especially if you're using bottled nutrients, it is a good idea to flush your plants. Even if you do not flush your plants intentionally, you should still give your plants dechlorinated water during the last 10 days or so before harvesting.

Step 5: Cut Down Your Plants

In this step, you begin harvesting your plants by cutting all or part of them down. You will use shears or a pair of long-handled loppers for bigger plants. Some smaller plants can easily be cut down whole, but this will not be possible or practical with large plants. In the case of large plants, you will have to break them down into smaller, more manageable pieces. I recommend that you keep the pieces that you harvest as large as possible for the drying process if you have the space to do so.

To harvest an entire plant, cut it down at the base, just below the first set of branches. If you have enough room to hang the whole plant, I recommend doing so. Start with the top colas and then work your way down to the bottom of the plant. You may find that you want to leave the bottom to mature for a longer amount of time.

When cutting plants up to hang dry, use your hand pruners to cut one end of the stalk so as to

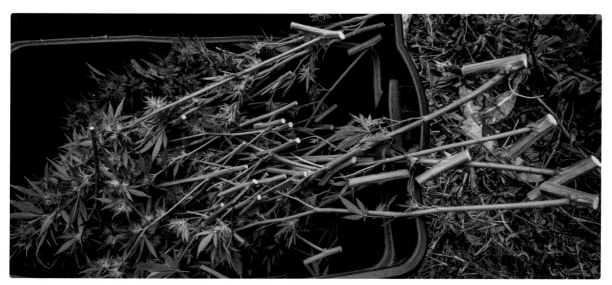

The plants shown here were harvested by cutting through the main stem a couple inches above and below each branch. This creates a J-shaped end or "hook" that you can use to hang the plants for drying.

leave a hook or "J" shape, about 2–3 inches (5–7.5 cm) above each branch (see the photo on page 169). It will make drying your crop a lot easier, as you can use this hook to help you hang and take down your branches from the string.

I recommend that you only harvest the plant material that you can process and hang in the amount of time that you have available. It is best not to leave harvested branches and plants for more than a few hours before trimming and hanging. If you have to do this, be sure to leave them in a cool place with good airflow. If at all possible, try to place them up off the ground.

Step 6: Trim Your Plants

At some point, you are going to need to remove the excess leaves from your flowers. Your buds will burn, taste, smell, and look better if you trim them. (Before drying, it is also a good idea to remove the big fan leaves from the plant).

There are a couple of approaches for trimming. You can trim your flowers when they are fresh, a process known as "wet trimming," or after they have dried, known as "dry trimming." You can even save trimming until the last minute, right before you use your buds (see "Storing Untrimmed Flowers" on page 188). Some growers also use machines. Machine-trimming can save you time, but it carries

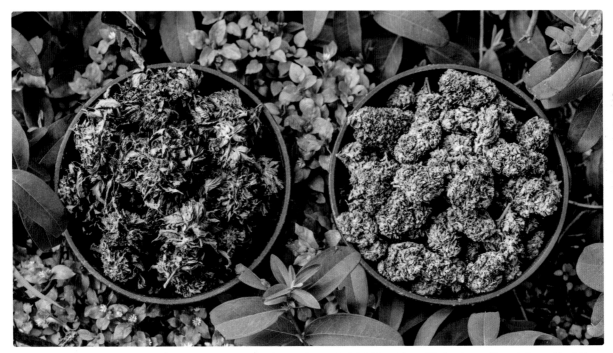

Trimming is the process of removing excess leaves from your buds. The container on the left holds untrimmed buds, whereas the container on the right holds trimmed buds.

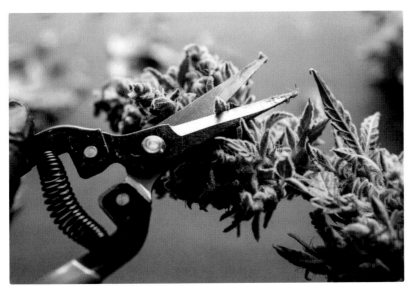
Trimming requires careful handling to avoid damaging the trichomes on your buds.

the risk of damaging your buds and causing the quality of your cannabis to suffer as a result. I will cover wet and dry trimming next.

No matter which approach you choose, note that trimming can take a long, long time—hours, days, weeks, even months—depending on the size of your harvest and if you have any help. Be sure to plan accordingly.

Wet versus Dry Trimming

There are benefits to both wet and dry trimming. Wet trimming is ideal if there is damage due to pests or mold on your flowers. It reduces the amount of plant material that you have to dry, which is ideal if you have limited space in your drying room, and it cuts down on the time it takes for your harvest to dry. It is also easier to trim your

flowers when they are fresh and you can break the plants down into smaller pieces.

Dry trimming lengthens dry times for your harvest slightly, but the leaves that you keep on the branches will protect the buds and trichomes throughout the drying process. Your flowers will be less likely to develop a hay smell, which happens when chlorophyll leaks from the cut leaves into the flowers when you wet-trim. You can also hang whole plants or bigger portions of plants and spend less time breaking plants apart before drying. Most important, keeping your plants as whole as possible for as long as possible protects the trichomes (and the terpenes contained within them) and keeps them intact longer, resulting in better-smelling and -tasting flowers.

I strongly advise you to dry-trim your buds. It is one of the big differences between how corporate and craft cannabis producers create their product, and the taste, smell, and quality of dry-trimmed buds is undeniable. As a home grower, you are going to end up with better-quality flowers when you make the decision to dry-trim. But, as always, the final decision is up to you and depends on your needs and constraints. You may even wish to try both approaches and compare the results.

Your Trimming Workspace

Set up a clean, cool, and well-lit area for your workspace with a comfortable chair and table. A bright light is crucial so that you can closely inspect your buds for signs of disease, damage, and mold. Overhead or movable lighting is best for this. Don't forget some music—enjoy this time and celebrate all your hard work!

There are a few tools that you'll need to keep yourself comfortable and make the process quicker and more efficient:

- Scissors or small handheld pruners
- Pruning shears

- Rubbing alcohol and a small jar (for cleaning your scissors and shears)
- Gloves made from a tight-fitting material, such as latex (optional)
- Containers or trays for your untrimmed buds, trimmed buds, trichomes, and other stray trimmings
- A trim container, also known as a trim bin (optional)—a specialized bin with a screen on the bottom that will separate and collect the trichomes that fall off your buds as you trim so that you can easily gather and store them for later use.

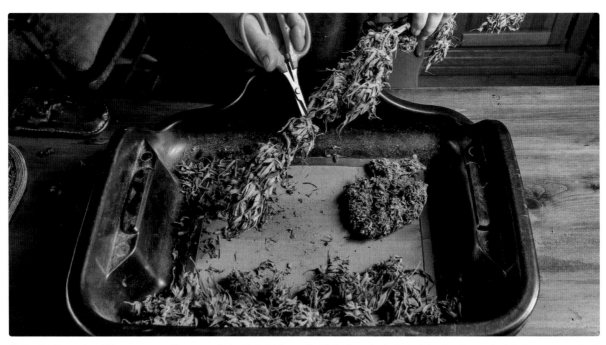

A trimming bin, such as this one, comes with a screen that collects trichomes that fall off your buds during trimming. It can also help keep you organized and comfortable when trimming for long periods of time.

How to Trim

If you did not take the fan leaves off when the plant was still alive, then you should do this first. Always remove the whole leaf stalk off the plant. Make sure to cut it down at the base (close to the stem) and get the whole petiole. If you leave part of the stem, there is a chance for mold to form in this spot. In most cases, the larger leaves that do not contain trichomes can be added back into your garden beds or put into the compost pile. Anything that looks off should be discarded or at least separated from the rest of the buds.

Whether you choose to wet- or dry-trim your plants, the trimming process is essentially the same. Manicure the buds by removing all the excess leaves that are protruding from the buds. Be careful not to cut into the buds as you remove the leaves. This will not only save you time, but it will inflict considerably less damage on the buds and their valuable trichomes. Trim away the full leaves as well as the single blades that are growing out from the buds. Your trimmed buds should preserve the size, shape, and structure of the flower. Make sure you do not cut into the flower; doing this will not only damage the bud itself, but it will lower the quality and damage the precious trichomes.

As you trim, be sure to save the trimmings, also known as "sugar shake." You will see that these small leaves will be covered in trichomes, and it

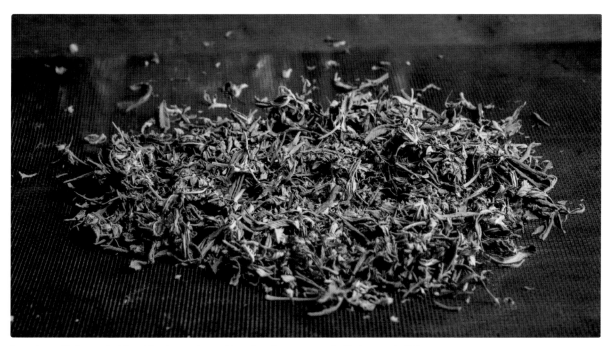

Sugar leaves that you collect from trimming can be used to make salves, creams, oils, tinctures, and edibles.

would be a shame not to put them to good use. They make great hash, edibles, and other items, such as salves and tinctures.

Every now and then, you will find that your scissors are coated in resin and need to be cleaned. Before wiping them with rubbing alcohol, be sure to scrape off the resin and save it for later use. This potent "scissor-hash" will give you a good buzz. After each trimming session, clean your scissors and pruners so they are ready to go for your next session.

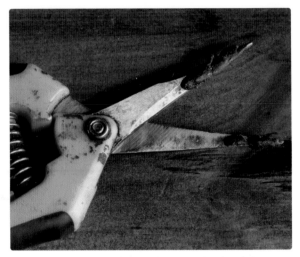

You can scrape off the resin on your trimming tools and use it for smoking, vaping, or other preparations.

HARVESTING TIPS & TRICKS

Be gentle. Any time you handle your buds, whether during harvesting, trimming, or de-fanning, always avoid being too aggressive or heavy-handed. Inexperienced trimmers (and especially those who use machines) can severely damage buds, which can seriously impact the final product. Go slowly when you are first learning to trim and take your time. You will become quicker and more efficient with experience.

Always be on the lookout for powdery mildew and gray mold. If you spot any, be sure to cut it all out and dispose of any affected material. Even a small amount of mold can travel throughout the entire bud during the drying process and ruin what would otherwise be good flowers. Be sure to inspect every branch and bud, making sure to look closely at the stalk and the center of each bud for discoloration, damage, mold, powdery mildew, or anything unusual. A bright, overhead light will be indispensable when examining your flowers.

Ask for help with trimming. Recruiting people to help you trim can get the job done a lot faster. Always be careful whom you invite to a trim party, and be sure to ask your helpers to avoid spreading the word about your harvest. Even though cannabis is now legal in a lot of areas, there is always the chance that people may want to steal what you have.

FAQS & TROUBLESHOOTING

Q: What should I do if my plants are not fully mature, but there is bad weather coming in?

A: This is a tricky question to answer because there are a lot of factors at play. What I would say is this: Look at the weather forecast, and get an idea of how long the inclement weather is going to last and what the conditions will be like after it passes. If the weather will be clear after a storm, it could be fine to leave your plants and harvest them at a later date. If the weather forecast is going to be bad for a number of days, it may be better to harvest a little early, rather than waiting and taking the risk of losing part of your harvest to mold or having the quality of your flowers suffer.

Q: What if my plants did not fully mature before the cold fall weather arrives?

A: There is most likely nothing that can be done to allow the plants to fully mature. If this happens to you, it may mean that the cultivars that you chose are not a good fit for your area. I always recommend harvesting your flowers, rather than letting them be ruined by cold weather and frost. It is better to harvest flowers that are a little immature than to let them spoil in your garden. In the future, remember that it is important to match the cultivars you grow to your growing region, and it may take some time and trial and error to figure out which ones work best for you.

Q: Will my buds really be lower quality if I decide to wet-trim my plants?

A: In my opinion, dry trimming creates a superior final product in terms of quality, smell, and taste. If you are new to growing, I recommend that you dry-trim and stick with that method. I have done my fair share of both, and I know many people who wet-trimmed for years, but say that they would never go back to dry trimming after switching and seeing the results. That said, do what makes sense to you and know that you can still obtain quality buds through wet trimming as well.

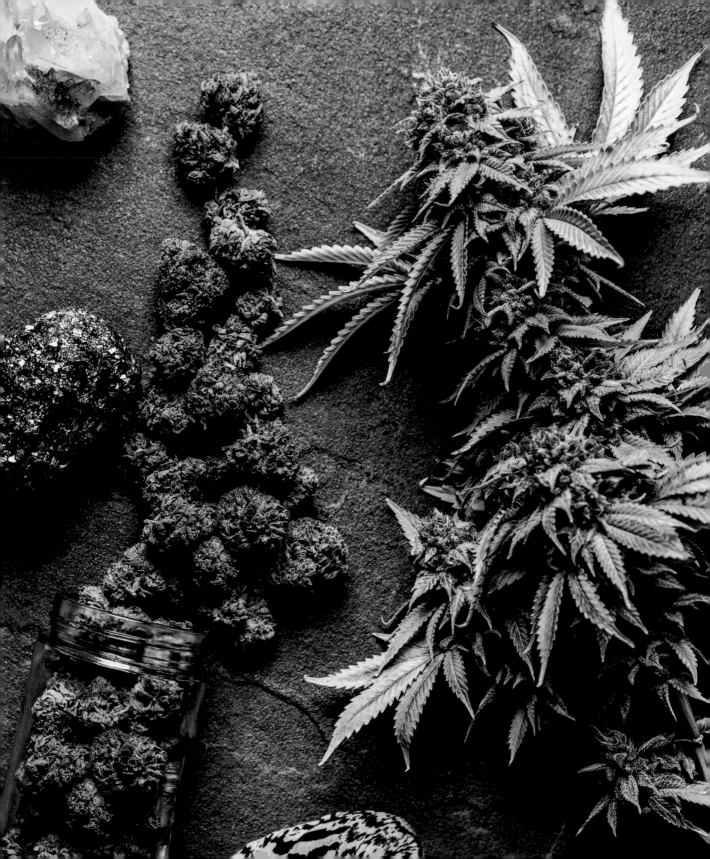

CHAPTER 11

< Drying & Curing >

The process of drying and curing is where the art and science of cannabis growing meet. They are the most important factors that determine whether you will have a high-quality final product. It is through proper drying and curing that your cannabis flowers truly become a thing of beauty. This process preserves and protects the valuable terpenes and cannabinoids, and, when done properly, they will give you the most beautiful-smelling and -tasting buds that you could imagine. This is where the time, dedication, practice, and experience of the grower can shine through. However, these are areas where many inexperienced growers make the most mistakes, causing the quality of their flowers to suffer tremendously. Knowing how to dry and cure your cannabis properly is crucial for preserving the potency and smell of your flowers for future use. This chapter will walk you through the entire process.

DRYING

As with all herbs, freshly harvested cannabis can and should be preserved for future use with drying. It is a critical step toward preserving your harvest and keeping it from spoiling. A properly dried cannabis flower will retain its potency, smell, and quality for your own personal enjoyment and medicinal needs. Plus, why would you put all that time into taking care of and growing your plants only to rush the drying process?

Setting Up a Drying Space

It is of utmost importance to have a plan for drying your flowers before you harvest your plants. The first step of that planning involves setting up a proper space for drying. You want to find an area that is on the cooler side and dark. It should have good airflow, and the temperature and humidity should remain steady.

The optimal temperature range to dry cannabis is 60°F–65°F (15°C–18°C), and optimal humidity levels are 55–60 percent. If your temperature

LEFT Properly drying and curing your buds will ensure that they retain much of their terpene profiles and remain flavorful and potent.

< 177 >

rises above 75°F (24°C), some of your terpenes can volatize and dissipate, never to be smelled or tasted again. If your humidity is too high, you run the risk of spoiling your flowers as they will not dry, and, conversely, if the humidity is too low, your flowers will dry too quickly and their taste and smell will suffer as a result.

There are a number of ways you can set up a drying space, but one of the easiest and most practical methods for the home grower is simply to string lines from which you can hang your plants upside down. A strong nylon string, mason line, or wire will work well for this. Make sure that the strings are securely fastened to a solid anchor

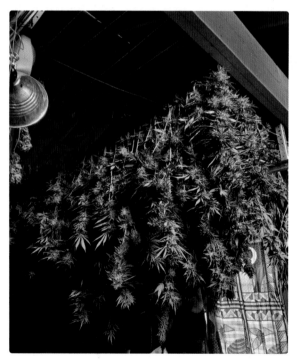

It is important for your drying space to be dark, have a stable temperature and humidity level, and allow for some airflow.

(your buds are going to be heavy!). Depending on your setup and the size of your harvest, you may want to string lines in multiple tiers.

After this is done, set up a thermometer and a hygrometer to monitor conditions in your drying space. It should be at the same level as your flowers when they are hanging. To help maintain good airflow, place an oscillating fan in the space, but avoid having the fan blowing air directly on your drying flowers. Moving air around the room as your buds dry will help moisture evaporate and prevent mold from forming.

It is a balancing act to maintain the correct environmental conditions in your drying room at all times. If you are in a northern climate, you may need to set up a small portable heater if the space is not already heated. In warmer climates, you may need a way to cool your room down, such as installing an air conditioner or opening a window or a door. For humid areas, a dehumidifier will help maintain the proper humidity.

Once you have set up your drying space, be sure you monitor it with a temperature and humidity gauge for a day or two to make sure that there are no wild fluctuations. The humidity may spike in your drying room right after you bring a lot of plants into it. This is fine for a day or two, but you want to make sure that it comes down to 60 percent within that time. Having a gauge that can record a minimum and maximum reading is ideal, as it will let you know what the conditions were in the room overnight and throughout the day.

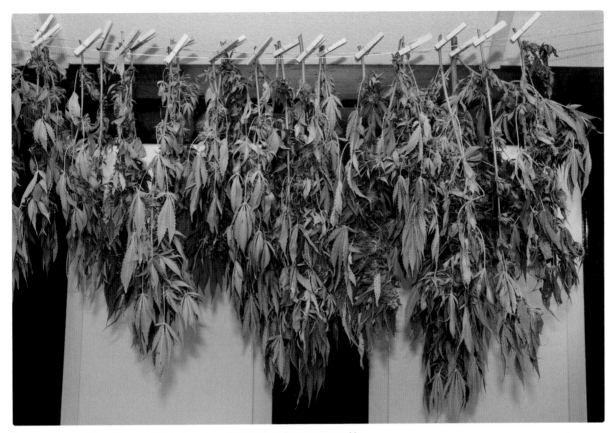
You can use many different household objects, such as clothespins, to hang your cannabis.

Hanging Your Plants

There are several ways to hang your plants. As mentioned in the last chapter (see page 170), you can cut the end of the plants' stems into a "hook" as you're harvesting. If this is not possible, you can hang the branches on a side bud or, if the branches are small, clothespins or paper clips may work. Feel free to get creative!

As you hang your buds on the lines, be sure to leave adequate space between each one so that air can circulate among the branches. I would recommend leaving 1–2 inches (2.5–5 cm) between the buds as they hang, making sure that they do not touch each other. As the drying process progresses, they will shrink and increase the space between the branches. This will limit the chances of mold forming and allow the buds to dry more evenly.

Some people will destalk (see page 183) and dry their buds on screens (see page 182). This is not my first choice, and I recommend that you hang whole plants and larger branches whenever possible. I find that buds placed on screens tend to dry too quickly, and their quality suffers as a result. This drying method also requires a bit more attention, as you need to stir the buds regularly to prevent flat spots from forming. However, drying screens do work well for smaller branches and the random buds that break off larger branches, so having a couple on hand is a good idea. There are a few different ways of drying your plants (see the sidebar on page 182 for more ideas). Try some of them and compare the results and record them in your plant journal. The most important thing is that you end up with a final product that you like.

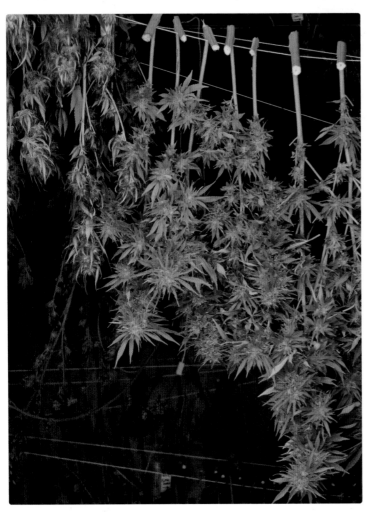

You can use the stems of the plants to hang the branches, especially if you cut the ends into a "J" shape (see page 169).

Drying Time Frame

You want to have your cannabis dry slowly. Not only will this preserve the quality of your flowers, but it will also allow you to retain many of the terpenes, making your cannabis taste, smell, and look much better than plants that dry too quickly. Ten to 14 days of drying time is ideal, but there are many factors that will determine how slowly your plants dry.

Generally speaking, the larger the plants (or pieces thereof), the longer they will take to dry. The same is true for the size of the buds; bigger buds mean slower drying times. The temperature, humidity, and whether these stay steady will also play a role. You can slow down the drying process considerably when you leave the buds on the stalks, as the buds continue to draw water from the stalks even as moisture evaporates from the buds themselves. If your flowers dry a little sooner than the 10–14-day time frame, that is fine. Just make sure they do not become super dry and crispy. It is better to bring them down off the line sooner and get them curing than leaving them to overdry.

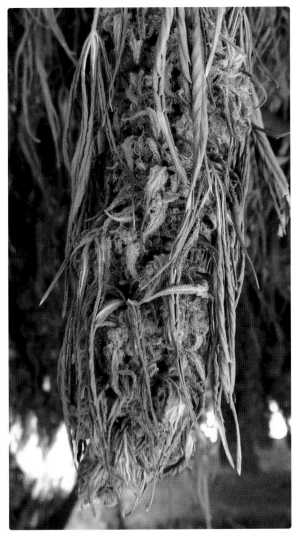

When your buds have finished drying, they will lose some of their bright green color and make a snapping sound when they are broken off the stem.

It is a good idea to check on your plants at least once a day as they dry. Because you should keep your drying space dark, you can turn on a light or use a flashlight to inspect your flowers. Look for signs of mold, and make sure that one area of your room is not drying more quickly or more slowly than another. It is a good habit to feel your buds throughout the drying process to get an idea of how they are drying. Don't squish them, and be gentle. Your sense of touch is key in this process. You may also want to move your fans, dehumidifiers, and heaters to different places to ensure that the plants are drying well and evenly. Inspecting your room does not have to be a long and intensive process, but be sure you are doing it regularly.

Your buds are ready to come down and transition into the curing process when the following happens:

- The buds are crispy on the outside.

- You hear a snapping sound when you bend one of the buds on the stalk. The bud may snap right off the branch. Be sure to test a few different-sized buds and stalks, since the smaller ones will dry first and the larger ones will take a little longer.

- Your harvest has spent at least 1 week or more under the ideal drying conditions described in this chapter.

ADDITIONAL DRYING METHODS

- Hang a small number of flowers on clothes drying racks or stands. For drying racks, you can hang the branches from each rung or drape them across the rack in a horizontal fashion.

- Clothes hangers work well for hanging flowers. You can hang the plants from the end of the stem or a branch or pin them onto the hanger with a clothespin or paper clip.

- Trellis netting offers you many options for hanging a lot of flowers. You can hang the branches from many different locations on the netting or create netting with multiple levels. Trellis netting will let you easily hang cannabis from the ceiling or wall.

- Cut your flowers from the branches and put them in the hanging mesh bins or trays.

- Use drying screens or window screens. Place the branches or buds on the screens and be sure to stir or rotate them at least once or twice a day to prevent the sides of the buds that are resting against the screen from flattening. It is best to suspend the window screens to allow air to flow underneath them. You can also put these screens on a table, propping up the sides of the screens with a stack of books, bricks, or wood to create airflow beneath the buds.

- If you do not have a dedicated space for drying, a closet or cardboard box is a potential option. If you're using a large cardboard box, punch holes in each side of the box, thread strings through those holes, and tie knots to create lines to hang your branches from. You can then close the top of the box, opening it a few times a day to allow air exchange, or simply leave it open.

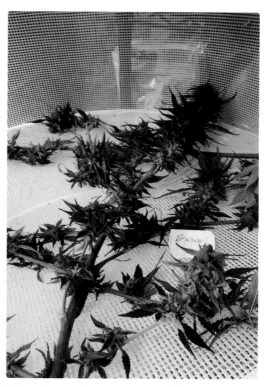

This small immature branch broke off in a storm and is now being dried in a hanging basket dryer. Drying baskets and racks work well for branches and buds of this size.

Destalking

Destalking is the process of removing the buds from the stalks. This is also called "bucking." This can be done between the drying and curing stages or after the curing stage when you are getting ready to seal up and store your buds. (The advantage of the former option is that buds without stalks will take up less space in your curing containers.) It is easiest to separate the buds from the stalks with a pair of scissors or pruning shears. The leftover stalks can be put into the compost pile.

It is at this point that many growers will grade their flowers by size, separating the large and medium buds from the small ones. Growers will also separate the immature buds, also known as "minging" or "larf" buds, to be used for hash or products such as oils, tinctures, and edibles. I recommend that you organize and grade your flowers in this manner if you have the time and desire to do so. It is always nice to have your top-quality flowers separated and easily available to access as your own personal "head stash."

If you do your destalking over a screen or a container (or "trim bin"), save all the trichomes or resin heads that have fallen off the buds and sifted through the screen. These trichomes are commonly known as *kief*, a form of dry sift hash. This potent material would otherwise be lost and can be used for smoking, vaping, or for a number of medicinal products, such as edibles, tinctures, or oils.

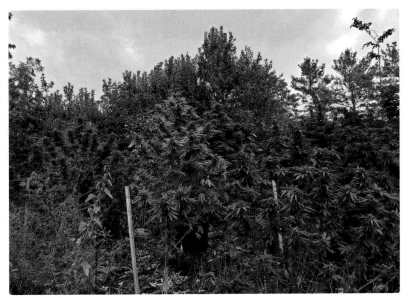

The flowers on these plants are almost ready to harvest. I prefer to take all the fan leaves off a plant when it is still in the ground. What better way to enjoy a beautiful fall day?

CURING

Curing involves drying your flowers for a second time over an extended period of time. It can last anywhere from a couple of weeks to several months. Why is it important to cure cannabis? After the initial drying stage, your buds will feel dry, but deep within the buds and stalks, there is still a little moisture. The curing process brings that moisture out from the center of the flower through a process called "sweating" and evenly distributes it over time. Some moisture will evaporate as well. Chlorophyll and starches will degrade, which enhances the taste and smell of your flowers.

This process is what takes your cannabis to another level. It accentuates the taste, smell, and quality of your buds. Many growers do not cure their harvest (or at least do not do it well), but once you experience the quality of well-cured cannabis flowers, you will never skip this step!

How to Cure

Curing is done in a slow fashion, over time, in a sealed container. I recommend curing your buds for a minimum of 1 month, but 1½–2 months is ideal.

Some growers will leave their buds sealed in a container for longer periods before opening them up. This allows the buds to lightly ferment, imparts a very sweet smell, and brings out the subtle flavors of the buds. But you want to be careful in doing this. If you leave the jars or totes sealed for too long in low-oxygen conditions, your buds will be susceptible to mold. Long-term curing is an advanced approach and one that I recommend that you try with a small amount of your harvest to gain experience before using this technique with your whole stash. If you're a beginner, I suggest following the steps listed to cure your buds.

CURING AT A GLANCE

1. Check your curing environment.

2. Put your buds into a sealed jar or a large container, such as a tote.

3. Sweat and "burp" your buds. This involves keeping them in a sealed container and opening the lids of your containers for a couple of minutes a couple of times a day to release built-up moisture or gases and allow fresh air to enter.

4. After a minimum of 4 weeks and up to 2 months, your buds will be ready to use in whatever way you desire.

Step 1: Check Your Curing Environment

It is best to cure your flowers in a room that has a humidity level of 50–55 percent and temperatures in the range of 60°F–64°F (15°C–18°C). Note that these conditions are slightly different from the ideal drying conditions outlined above. If your environment is too warm, you risk causing some of the precious terpenes to dissipate, leading to a loss of aroma. And if your environment is too dry, your buds will dry out too much and too quickly, causing the overall quality to suffer as well.

Step 2: Place Your Flowers in Containers

To begin curing, you need to put your buds into a sealed jar or container. It is best to use glass whenever possible. For larger harvests, plastic totes or fiber drums work well. Keep the containers in a dark place, away from the light. Be careful not to squish or pack your flowers too tightly.

Step 3: Open Your Containers

For the first 1 or 2 weeks, you will open the lids of your containers for 2–3 minutes, twice a day, to allow the moisture to evaporate, new air to enter the container, and off-gases to dissipate. This is called "burping." You will need to burp your containers less frequently as your buds continue curing. Use your sense of touch to monitor the moisture level of your buds as they cure, and your sense of smell to notice the changes as curing progresses. After 2 weeks or so, you may only need to open the jars every few days to exchange the air and check how the buds are doing. Eventually, you will notice that there is no off-gas buildup or a "seal" being broken when you open your jars. If using totes, the seal will not be as tight as the seal of a glass container. This is fine. Just make sure the humidity and temperature in your curing container fall within the optimum range. You may find that you do not need to open the lids and burp the totes nearly as much as you would need to if you were using glass jars.

There is a delicate balance between the buds being too wet and too dry. If there is too much moisture, you may need to leave the lid off for 1 or 2 hours or until you feel that the outside layer of the bud is noticeably drier than before. You can also remove your buds from the container and place them back in, adding the buds in the top layer first. This allows the bottom layer of buds, where moisture is often more prevalent, to move to the top of the container.

Step 4: Check for Signs of Curing

You will know that the curing process is taking place when there is a beautiful smell wafting from your buds. The buds will also feel drier. Well-dried and -cured cannabis flowers have a sweet smell and taste and will not be harsh when you smoke or vaporize them. They should burn smoothly, produce a nice white ash, and stay lit. Poorly dried and cured flowers will have little or no smell or may even smell like hay, and, when burned, they will leave behind a dark, crumbly, black ash.

PROPER STORAGE

After your buds have had ample time to cure, you are now ready to store them for future use. There are a few factors you will need to consider to make sure your buds will stay fresh.

Options for Containers

The options listed below can be used for both long-term storage (more than 6 months) and short-term storage (6 months or less). Depending on how much plant material you have, some options will work better than others.

Glass jars: Storing your cannabis in glass jars is your best option for preserving the quality, smell, and potency of your buds. Glass does not off-gas or react negatively to resin. When using jars, fill them to the top, but do not pack the jars too tightly or cram and squish the buds. Glass is always my first recommendation for storage, but if you have a very large harvest, it may not be possible to use glass exclusively.

Oven bags: Oven bags can also be a good choice and one that I would recommend over resealable bags (mentioned next). You can usually pick them up at your local butcher shop or online.

They are made with a food-grade plastic that is thicker than the type used for most storage bags.

Resealable food storage bags: There are many companies that make plastic resealable bags. They come in many sizes and can work well for keeping your flowers fresh for future use. One disadvantage to this option is that plastic can off-gas and potentially negatively interact with the resin from your buds if used for long-term storage.

Vacuum sealer: Vacuum sealers will let you take all the air out of a specialized storage bag and seal your buds inside. You want to make sure that you get as much oxygen out of the bag as possible to best preserve your buds. These work well for both short- and long-term storage. The only downside to vacuum sealing is that once you open up a bag, you cannot reseal it.

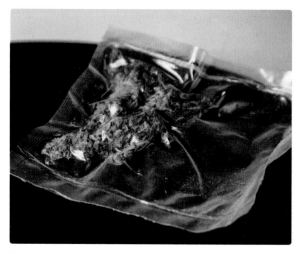

Vacuum-sealed bags can preserve buds for long periods of time.

Storing Cured Buds

You want to make sure that your buds are stored in a cool, dark place, ideally at 39°F–46°F (4°C–8°C) and out of direct sunlight. The humidity level should fall in the range of 55–63 percent humidity, both inside your container and in the place where you will keep the container. Stored in an environment like this, your cannabis will be in great condition for a year or more.

It is also acceptable to store your cannabis at room temperature. Cannabis stored at room temperature out of direct light will last for almost a year before you start to see signs of degradation, such as a loss of color and aroma. It will still be in decent condition as long as it has been dried and cured properly and it has not gone moldy. It will be perfectly fine to use for much longer. It may just lose some of its potency, smell, and visual appeal.

Many people do not recommend storing your flowers in the freezer because you run the risk of damaging the precious trichomes when you handle frozen flowers. However, if you know that you are not going to be using your flowers for 8 months or more, freezing is an option to consider. It is best to have your flowers a little on the drier side to prevent freezer burn, and do not touch, move, or squish them while they're in the freezer. When you take them out of the freezer, be sure to let them warm to room temperature before opening the bag and handling the buds. The best way to do this is to set the buds on a countertop to defrost at room temperature. Vacuum-sealed bags are the best for freezer storage as the removal of oxygen from the bags should prevent freezer burn.

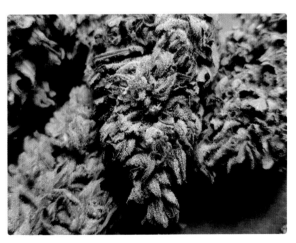

These dried and cured B67 buds are ready for use. They can be trimmed further or used as they are now.

HUMIDITY CONTROL PACKETS

There are a couple of products on the market that you can use to maintain the ideal humidity level inside your jars or bags. Integra and Boveda are companies that make two-way humidity-control packs. If your buds are too dry, they will release moisture, and if they are too wet, they will take in moisture. These products were made for the tobacco and cigar industries and are being adopted by the cannabis industry as well.

While humidity control packets work well for long-term storage, many growers do not like to use them, as they interrupt the slow drying process of the curing phase. I advise you to try them out if you want to and make up your own mind.

Storing Untrimmed Flowers

If you've chosen to dry-trim your buds (page 170), you have the option of storing them with most of the leaves (except the fan leaves) intact. There are a few reasons that this can be a good idea. First, the extra leaves help to protect the buds by shielding the trichomes and helping them stay intact if your buds get squished or bumped in the bag or jar. Second, by keeping them untrimmed, you do not need to cut and manipulate the buds as much, which prevents terpenes from dissipating and keeps your flowers smelling better for longer. Although untrimmed flowers do not have the same visual appeal as well-manicured flowers, you can rest assured that under the leaves are potent, intact trichomes, just waiting to unleash their effects onto its user. It won't take long to do a final trim on individual buds just before you use them, and remember to save that sugar shake for your edibles, tinctures, and topical products.

FAQS & TROUBLESHOOTING

Q: **What do I do if my drying space is not ideal in terms of all the parameters laid out in this chapter?**

A: You will simply have to make the most of whatever space you have available to you. Having your drying space on the cooler side is better than having it on the warmer side. Slightly higher humidity is better than a super-dry environment (but make sure the humidity is no higher than 65 percent). Pay attention to how your harvest dries and cures under the conditions that you have, and make notes in your plant journal on how you can improve the following year.

Q: **My buds are too dry and crumbly. Is there anything I can do?**

A: If your buds are too dry, you will need to rehydrate them. You can try adding a humidity pack (see sidebar above). An old school way of combating this problem is by using a few rinds of a citrus fruit, such as a lemon, a lime, or a grapefruit. Remove any wet parts from the inside of the rind. Equally space out the rinds in the container with your buds. Depending on the amount of cannabis you have, you will put in more or fewer rinds. The peel from half a lemon should be more than enough for a 16-ounce (470-ml) jar; divide the peel into four equal-size pieces and place in different locations inside the jar. (This works with a tortilla as well.) Leave the rinds in there for a couple of hours (or overnight if your cannabis is extremely dry), and monitor the moisture content by using your sense of touch. You should be able to feel a change in the buds as they soak up some of the moisture from the rind. If you happen to leave the rinds in the jar for too long, just leave the lid off or the bag open until your cannabis reaches the desired moisture content.

There are also other ways to rehydrate using a plastic tote with a lid and water. Put a bowl or tray of water at the bottom of the tote. Place your jars with the lids off or in an open bag into the tote, and close the lid. This creates an environment that allows the dry buds to soak up some of the moisture in the air. Be careful not to leave them for too long in this environment and check them consistently.

Q: What do I do if my buds still feel too moist after drying?

A: If your buds are still too moist, you need to let them dry longer. They may take anywhere from a couple of hours to an extra day or two, if they are very wet. Check them consistently and be sure to use your sense of touch. If you

have a small hygrometer available to you, that will also help you monitor the buds.

Q: Can I use a dehydrator to dry my buds quickly?

A: Yes, you can, but *it is not a good idea.* You will lose a lot of your terpenes and the smell of your cannabis when you dry too quickly or dry at too high a temperature. The resulting cannabis will be poor quality and will not taste, smell, or smoke well. The slower you can dry your cannabis, the better. Don't cut corners with this process!

Q: Can dried cannabis go bad? How do I tell if my cannabis is past its prime or if I stored it incorrectly?

A: Cannabis can certainly go bad if it has too much moisture and is sealed away too soon. Excess moisture means you run the risk of it growing mold, and if this happens, you will need to discard your buds. Cannabis should last at least 6–8 months before you notice or experience any loss in potency or visual appeal. If it does not last this long, you may need to make changes in your drying, curing, and storage process the next time around. Even when stored properly and with the correct moisture levels, your buds will begin to fade in color, lose their potency, and look less appealing over time. The cannabis is still fine to use; it just may lack the quality that it once had. Eventually, the cannabinoids will degrade naturally from THC or CBD to CBN (which can be very helpful as a sleep aid).

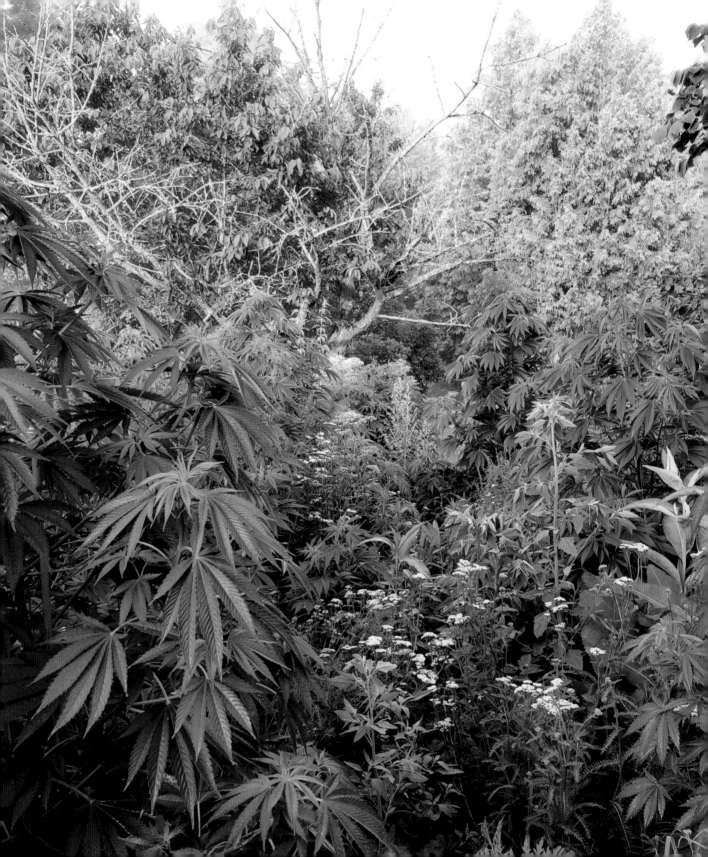

CHAPTER 12

< Planning Next Year's Garden >

There is an incredible and fulfilling feeling that comes after a successful growing season and a bountiful harvest. All the time, energy, hard work, care, and attention that you have given to your plants has paid off. With the turning of earth's seasons, you, too, are beginning to wrap up the season as well. This is a time for celebration and also a time for reflection—to look back, revisit your garden and your plants in your mind's eye, and start to bring some of the many lessons that you learned into your consciousness. While you celebrate, you can start to reflect on all that you learned over the course of the season. In this chapter, you will learn what you can do to process your experiences, to wrap up your year, and to plan for the next one.

END-OF-SEASON MAINTENANCE

You have finished your season, and are now ready to take it easy and perhaps enjoy some of the cannabis that you grew this past year, but before you put your tools away, you'll need to take care of some things first.

Any plant material that you are not going to use or make medicine from, should either go directly back into your beds to decompose over the winter or be put into your compost pile. This includes leaves, stems, stalks, plant material strained from oils or tinctures, and hash water. Some people will even chip or shred their cannabis stalks and add them back into their garden beds as mulch.

There are a couple of reasons for this. Returning plant matter to your garden is a regenerative practice. It closes a loop. Your plants have drawn a lot of nutrients from the soil and stored them in their living tissue. When you put some of this plant material back into the garden beds, you are

LEFT A snapshot of my garden in early summer. You can see many medicinal plants growing and thriving together. I like to greet the sunrise and a new day by enjoying a morning tea in this space.

< 191 >

putting some of those nutrients back into the soil. By putting this plant material back into your garden, you are also adding organic matter back into your soil.

It is always a good idea to go out into your garden, even in the off-season, and spend some time noticing and feeling the energy during this season. Tune into the land, the soil, and nature. Observe both the outer and inner worlds and take some time to relax, unwind, and connect with this space. Maybe even enjoy one of your favorite flowers in this place that provided so much for you. Honor and respect this space, this land, and this soil, and it will continue to provide for you and your plants long into the future.

TIP: If you produced some seeds, you can spend some time throughout the winter months separating them from the flower and starting to organize and catalog them for future planting. Perhaps there are people in your community you could give some to or trade for another cultivar to try. Share the seeds and share the love.

Cover Crops

Cover crops, also called green manure, serve a number of purposes, including boosting soil fertility; adding organic matter and nutrients back into the soil; and protecting it from drying out, erosion, and damage from rain. They outcompete

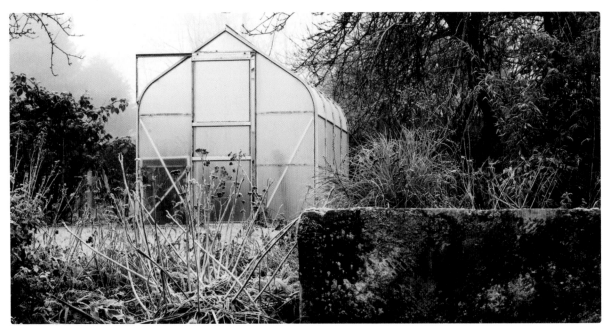

Winter is a time of rest for both you and your garden, but be sure to spend time here during this time so that you can experience this place from another perspective and observe how the change of the seasons impacts your growing space.

and smother weeds as well. If you're looking for an additional gardening project that can also benefit your soil, I recommend working with cover crops.

Cover crops are typically planted and grown in the shoulder seasons before you have planted or after you have harvested your cannabis. For example, you may choose to plant a winter-hardy cover crop in the fall after you have harvested your buds. In the early spring, this crop will come up and grow until you are ready to plant your new cannabis.

Some of the more commonly used plants as cover crops include the following:

Buckwheat: Buckwheat grows quickly and smothers weeds. It can do well in nutrient-poor soils, makes phosphorus more available, and harbors beneficial insects. It is killed by frost.

Dichondra: *Dichondra* spp. are perennial cover crops that are often grown at the same time as cannabis to help cover the soil, prevent it from drying out, and protect it from erosion. It also helps to smother weeds competing with your cannabis. This plant can spread, especially in warmer areas, so it may be best suited for planting in your pots or container gardens, depending on your local climate. In colder regions, it will die off from the cold temperatures.

Legumes: Legumes capture nitrogen from the air and deposit it into the soil. Some common legumes are red clover, hairy vetch, field peas and cowpeas, and alfalfa. Most will harbor beneficial insects as well as offer other benefits unique to each individual plant, such as protecting the soil from the heat of the sun and attracting pollinators to the garden.

Oats: Oats are a good weed suppressor and add organic matter to the soil. It takes up and holds soluble nitrogen, conditions topsoil, and attracts beneficial insects. It is killed by frost.

Sorghum: Sorghum helps to open up the subsoil, takes up and holds soluble nitrogen, and suppresses weeds. It is killed by frost.

Winter rye: Winter rye germinates and grows quickly, it's winter-hardy, and it helps with weed suppression. It also conditions topsoil and attracts beneficial insects.

When choosing your plants, it is important to know why these plants will benefit your particular garden and to know how long they will be growing for. Will they die when frost and cold weather arrive? Will they overwinter and grow again in the spring? Will you remove them to make room for your cannabis, or will you grow them alongside your cannabis? If you need to remove your cover crop, will you chop it down, cover it with occultation tarps, or rely on the weather to kill it off? These are all good questions to ask yourself as you plan and look for ways to integrate cover crops into your garden.

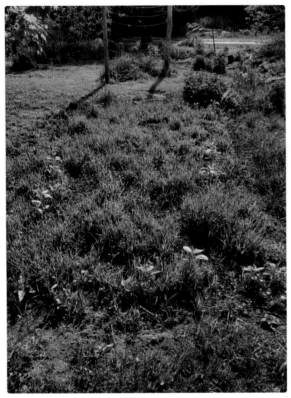

In early spring, I plant a mixture of oats, cowpeas, broad beans, red clover, alfalfa, and daikon radish as cover crops.

REFLECTIONS ON THIS YEAR'S GARDEN

Growing anything, whether it is ornamental flowers, vegetables, herbs, or cannabis, can be addicting. Once you nurture a plant through an entire season, you almost always want to do it again. Before you have even wrapped up drying and curing your flowers from this year, you may find yourself thinking ahead to the next season. *What new plants will I grow? Which ones will I grow again? What did I learn from my experiences this year? What changes will I make to improve, based on the lessons I learned this year?* The list of questions goes on and on.

Relive Your Growing Season

The key to answering these questions is to reflect on the many things that you learned in your current season and the things that you may want to change or do differently next season. As you begin to look back, I'd like you to visualize your most recent growing season, from the time you planted your first seeds to the present moment, trying to conjure up the images and memories, using all your senses. By reliving the growing season in your mind, you can continue to learn from the entire experience and sometimes even learn something that you were not consciously aware of beforehand. I have practiced this exercise for many years and continue to be amazed at the things that I can pick up on and learn from this simple meditative experience.

Begin by envisioning how different times of the day feel on your skin throughout the season—the cool early mornings of spring, the hot heat of the midday sun, a summer rain shower, the cool fall nights. Now, move to your sense of smell and imagine all the scents that drifted on the breeze—the smell before a rainstorm or the scent of your flowers or the soil at your feet. Now, shift your focus to your ears and listen to the sounds of the birds or frogs that live near you, perhaps the sounds of the crickets or buzzing insects during

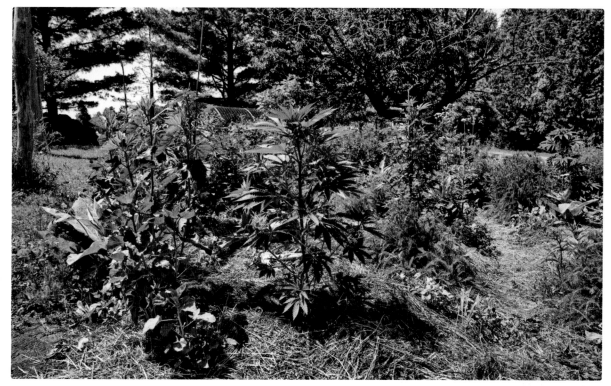

Taking the time to relive your growing season can help you learn more about the plants you grew, your garden, its needs, and its special quirks. This information will serve you well when you make plans for next year.

the long days of summer. Lastly, as you breathe in, use your sense of taste. What does the air feel like, what did the plants or flowers that grew among your cannabis plants taste like? Maybe there were some vegetables that you grew and ate this year.

It may be easiest to do this exercise with your eyes closed, but however you complete it, take your time and really re-create the many experiences you had this past year. Pay attention to anything that comes to you out of the blue. There may be something in these thoughts for you to learn from. You can do this inside your house or apartment, but if you can do it outside in your garden, that is even better.

Write It Down

Earlier in the book, I talked about the importance of keeping a plant journal. Now is the time to bring this journal out again. Flip through the pages, read your notes, and review any sketches that you made. When you get to the end of the journal, write down the following headings, using a blank sheet of paper for each one:

- **Celebrations:** Use this page to list and describe what went well this year.

- **Cultivar Notes:** What stands out to you about each plant you grew last year? Did it flower early or late? Was it resistant to pests or diseases? How did the flower turn out after the drying and curing process?

- **Lessons Learned:** Use this page to describe any challenges you had and what you would do differently to address them.

- **Notes on Soil:** Is there something you would like to add to your soil for next year? This is also a great place to list the soil amendments and teas that worked well.

You can also add separate pages for notes on insects, breeding, yield, pests and diseases, tolerances to different conditions, or nutrient deficiencies.

Looking Ahead

Once you have taken some time to reflect and make some notes on last year's garden, it will be time to let some of the lessons you've learned inform your decisions for next year's garden.

In your journal, create four more headings, using a new page for each one:

- **Next Year's Garden:** What do you want to accomplish next year? Are there any new growing methods that you want to try?

- **Future Planning:** What do you need to do in order to be ready for the growing season? Are there any tools and equipment that need maintenance? Make a list of these items and brainstorm ideas for any tools you'd like to acquire before next year.

- **Cultivar Selection:** What cultivars would you like to grow next year?

- **Next Year's Growing Schedule:** Sketch out the next growing season on a week-to-week or month-to-month basis. What are the things that you need to accomplish during each step?

As you reflect, you may find that your connection to your flowers is much deeper than it was in the past. Take this time to let the lessons sink in, and to celebrate this new relationship you have with this plant (or a deeper relationship, if this is not your first time growing). Feel proud of all you accomplished. Share some gratitude, and give thanks. Before you know it, you will be planting seeds and the cycle will begin again.

FAQS & TROUBLESHOOTING

Q: **How should I store tools and equipment that I'm not using during the winter?**

A: I recommend that you clean and sanitize all your tools with rubbing alcohol or hydrogen peroxide and then store them in a dry place, away from the elements. Some of your larger tools, such as shovels and buckets, can be left in a garage or another covered, unheated area. More delicate equipment, such as thermometers and lights, would be best stored indoors in an organized fashion so that they are out of the way but easy to locate when you need them for the next growing season.

Q: **This year's garden didn't turn out as planned, and my harvest didn't meet my expectations. How can I do better and be better prepared next year?**

A: First off, don't treat your results like a failure. Nothing is a failure, provided that you learn from the experience. Choose to look at it in a way that allows you to see and understand the lessons that you learned. Identify the mistakes that you made and the ways that you will improve and incorporate what you learned into the next growing season. Use the prompts and activities in this chapter to review your growing season and take notes on the improvements that you will incorporate into the following season. Make sure you write this information down so it is easily accessible when you need it. Growing cannabis is not always easy, and it takes time to become proficient at it. Don't give up. There is always next year, and you can always try again.

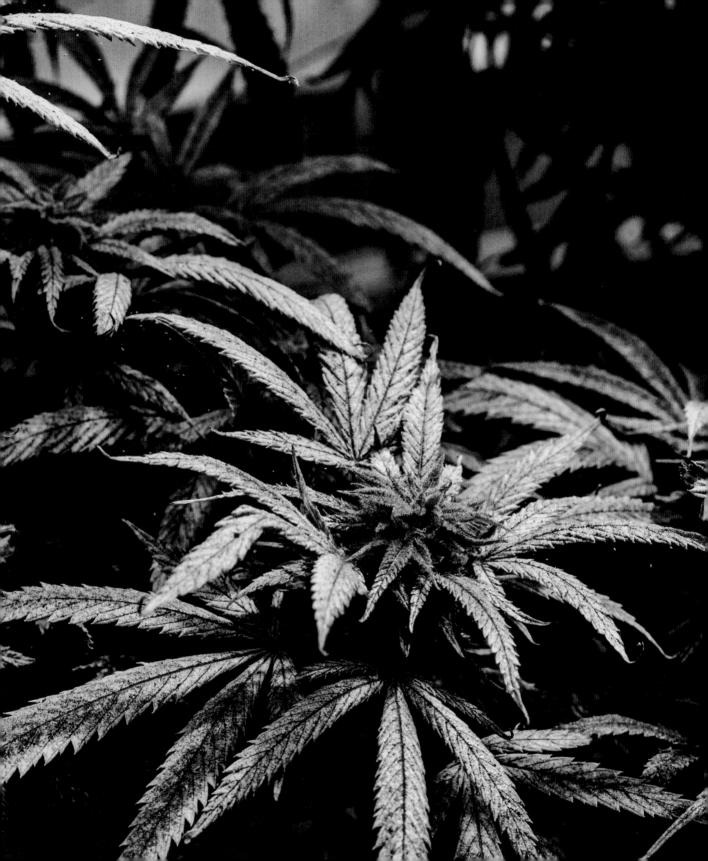

CHAPTER 13

< Common Pests, Diseases & Nutrient Imbalances >

This chapter will help you learn to detect the subtle and sometimes not-so-subtle clues about your plants' health. The information here will serve as a reference for diagnosing pests, diseases, and nutrient imbalances. Any grower who has been working with plants for more than a few years has had to deal with these issues. If they happen to you, think of them as a rite of passage on your growing journey.

DEVELOPING AN IPM PROTOCOL

Integrated pest management (IPM) describes a collection of practices that are used to detect, diagnose, and remediate any pests that visit your garden.

IPM protocols can include but are not limited to the following:

- Daily scouting and observation of your plants, both in terms of the garden as a whole and in minute detail, such as looking at the undersides of leaves with a jeweler's loupe

- Planning and managing your garden for optimal health

- Monitoring and identifying beneficial and detrimental insects in your garden

- Properly identifying pests, diseases, and nutrient imbalances in your garden

- Using organic sprays and natural repellents

- Introducing and attracting beneficial insects that prey on pests

- Using natural products to control pests, including microbial pesticides, fungicides, and more

LEFT The yellowing leaves on this cannabis plant are a result of a spider mite infestation (see page 209). Pests like these can quickly get out of control, especially in indoor environments.

< 199 >

- Observing and evaluating the effectiveness of your treatment measures

- Getting an experienced grower to give you a second opinion or to verify your diagnosis, treatment, and outcomes

Rather than having you react to pests as they emerge and focusing on short-term strategies, an IPM protocol encourages you to adopt a preventive mind-set. Before you think about controlling or eliminating a problem in your garden, ask yourself why this issue is happening in the first place. What is your garden lacking? What could you have done differently to avoid this situation? By looking at your garden in this manner, you will think of solutions that can resolve the issue at hand and also keep it from happening again in the future, ideally without the need to always rely on a spray or insecticide product.

For example, if aphids (see page 210) have shown up in your garden, instead of running for the spray bottle, ask yourself why they have appeared at this time and place. Are there any beneficial insects that can feed on the aphids? If so, how can you bring them to your garden? Can you cultivate a more diverse selection of plants to attract these insects and avoid future aphid infestations?

Practicing this type of critical thinking, the art of questioning, and looking deeply at each situation that arises will not only make you better prepared to deal with any challenge but also make you more resilient, adaptable, and flexible when facing future problems.

Learning to Look Closely

Every IPM protocol begins with careful and consistent observation of your plants. Once you have a baseline for what a healthy plant looks like, you will be better equipped to notice when its health has become compromised. The quicker you can spot pests, diseases, or nutrient imbalances of any kind, the quicker you will be able to deal with them and bring your plants back to health.

Here are some warning signs that something may be wrong:

- **There is discoloration in the leaves, stems, and flowers.** This may be a symptom of a nutrient deficiency or a pest issue.

- **The other plants in your garden look unhealthy.** If there is a nutrient deficiency, it might affect your entire garden. Some pests that attack cannabis might target other plants in your garden or spread easily from one plant to another.

- **There is damage from insects on leaves and stems.** Look closely at your plants for signs of insects feeding on your plants. If there are signs of feeding, find the insect that is causing the damage and identify the species. Once you know the species that is causing the damage, you can then develop a strategy to deal with it.

- **There are signs of mold on your leaves or flowers, or your plant is wilting, even after watering.** Be on the lookout for mold, powdery mildew, wilting, and anything that stands out and does not look healthy. These could be symptoms of disease.

If one of your plants is sick, this does not mean that all your plants will suffer. Different cannabis cultivars will show varying resistances to pests and disease, and not all cannabis plants will behave, grow, or require the same care or the same amount of certain nutrients. This is where your ability to select and get to know specific cultivars will be helpful.

> **TIP:** Yellow sticky surface traps can offer you a snapshot of the insects that visit your indoor garden and allow you to see potential pests before your plants show signs of a serious infestation. Sticky traps can also give you an idea of how many or how few of the insects there are, so you can tell the difference between a minor outbreak and a full-blown infestation.

Promoting Plant Health

One of the most important goals of your IPM protocol is to support and strive for super-healthy plants. The best defense against pests and diseases is strong plants that have all the nutrients they need and grow in the best environment possible. Healthy plants will fend off many pests and diseases and not allow them to take hold, whereas stressed and compromised plants will be more susceptible to them. Your observant care and close attention to your plants at every stage of growth from seedling to harvest will keep your plants disease- and

Issues with your plants can be tricky to diagnose. For example, discolored leaves can be a sign of a nutrient deficiency, as is the case here, but leaves might also yellow or die back naturally during flowering.

pest-free. Pay attention and give love to every member of your garden.

This is especially important if you are growing indoors without access to living soil or opportunities to attract beneficial insects. Indoor growers can purchase beneficial insects that can help control specific pests. Keep your growing area clean, make sure there is adequate airflow through the garden, and watch the temperature and humidity levels to prevent many pests and diseases when growing inside. A clean grow room is a happy and pest-free grow room!

Harness Biodiversity

There are several ways to ensure that your garden can fend off pests on its own. Many of these suggestions involve cultivating cannabis alongside other plants.

Companion plants: Having a wide array of various flowering plants will help to attract beneficial insects that feed on pests (see page 207). The more biodiversity in your garden, the better. Some good companion plants to consider are listed on page 46.

Trap plants: Many plants can be used to draw pests away from your cannabis plants. We call these "trap plants." They can be planted as a barrier around your garden or interspersed with your cannabis plants. Different plants will attract different insects. For example, broad beans entice spider mites, thrips, and whiteflies, while aphids and whiteflies favor nasturtiums (and will often completely cover their stems).

Banker plants: Banker plants attract and host beneficial insects that will feed on some of the specific plants in your garden. They are commonly used in greenhouses (many growers will cultivate about two banker plants per acre), but can be used in your outdoor gardens as well. Banker plants are easy to grow and do not affect the local ecosystem in a negative way. A quick internet search will yield many results for examples of banker plants, the beneficial insects they host, and the pests those beneficial insects will prey on.

Choosing Treatments

Once you spot an issue, it is important to identify it and consider all your options before reacting to it. There are a number of preventive measures that can be taken to avoid these potential issues. However, sometimes this is not enough.

When an issue arises in my garden, I start by thinking of the least invasive and easiest ways to fix the problem. Can I change the environment? Add nutrients to the soil or use a foliar spray? Are there beneficial insects present in the garden, or could I order some from an insectary? If all else fails, then I will consider using a natural, organic spray.

When it comes to sprays, I never use harmful chemicals or pesticides. Even if they are approved for use in growing food or cannabis, they are not an

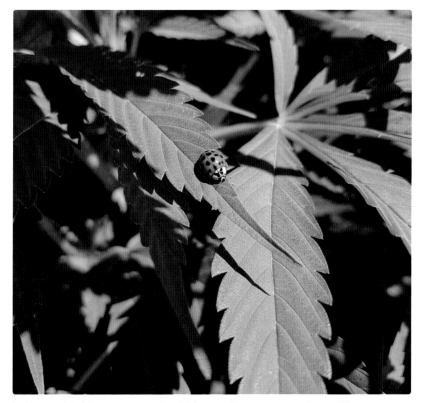
Ladybugs and their larvae are a good line of defense against many pests such as aphids.

When working with store-bought products, I recommend using the least amount possible that produces results. Start by using a little less than the recommended amount or the lower end of a recommended range. Because most products need to be mixed with water, you can instead add a little more water to create a slightly diluted solution. If the diluted mixture is ineffective, increase the dosage. It is also important to understand the life cycle of a particular insect to make sure that you are using a treatment at the most effective time, ideally before a new generation hatches.

After applying a product or homemade spray, monitor your plants to gauge its effectiveness. With homemade sprays, you will generally need to reapply every 4–7 days or so for a couple of weeks or until you see the desired results. It is also a good idea when using a new product or recipe to only spray a small portion of one plant and make sure it is not going to affect your plants negatively before applying it to your entire crop. Never spray your plants after they have begun to flower.

ethical choice for me because I do not want them coming in contact with my cannabis, especially when it will be used medicinally. There are recipes for homemade sprays in this book that can be very effective and are made from natural ingredients.

If you do not have access to the ingredients for these homemade solutions, you may want to consider purchasing a store-bought product. I recommend that you try to find ones that are made from natural ingredients and come with a certificate that they are approved for use in organic growing (see page 234 for organic certifying boards in your country).

Homemade Insecticidal Soap

What You Need

1 tablespoon castile soap (such as Dr. Bronner's)

1 cup (240 ml) olive oil or another vegetable oil

1 cup (240 ml) warm water

1. Add the soap to the oil and stir until thoroughly mixed. Then add 2 tablespoons of this mixture to the warm water and pour this into your spray bottle. You can mix more or less, depending on how much you need; just adjust the recipe. Before and during application to your plants, be sure to shake the bottle to prevent the solution from separating.

STORAGE: Any excess mixture of the oil and soap can be stored in a jar with a lid at room temperature for future use. When you are ready to use, mix it with water as noted in the recipe and apply.

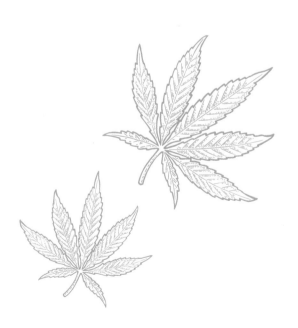

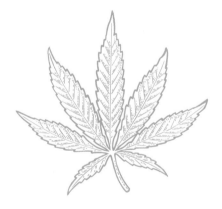

Pest Control Products

There are a few natural store-bought products and various biological controls that can help you fight pests. Biological controls are living organisms that are the natural enemies of various pests and diseases. However, for outdoor plants, note that even a botanical or biological preparation may have a negative impact or harm the lives of your allies—beneficial insects—so use them with caution.

Insecticidal soap: Insecticidal soap is a combination of soap, oil, and water and can be very effective at controlling the soft-bodied insects that do damage to your plants without killing helpful hard-bodied insects, such as ladybugs. You can purchase this product in stores as a ready-to-use solution or a concentrate that needs to be diluted with water. Follow the instructions on the label for mixing and application rates. You can also make your own insecticidal soap by following the recipe on page 204. Insecticidal soap should be sprayed directly onto pests above and below the leaves.

Microbial insecticides: Microbial insecticides use microorganisms, such as fungi, bacteria, or protozoa, as active ingredients to control various pests or diseases. Each microorganism targets a specific pest or condition, including powdery mildew and pests such as fungus gnats and thrips. Most are approved for organic use, and many of them can be mixed with water and either sprayed onto your plants or used as a soil drench. (A soil drench is a water-based solution that is added to the soil and delivers nutrients, fertilizers, or natural insecticides to the root zone of your plant.) Research the microorganisms and products that will be effective for the situation that you are dealing with. Be sure to follow the mixing instructions and application rates listed on each individual product.

Neem oil: This oil is made from the seeds and fruit of the neem tree, a type of evergreen. It has natural insecticide and fungicide properties and can be used preventively. Neem oil is generally applied on the leaves, but it can also work as a root drench to kill unwanted nematodes in soil.

To use, mix with warm water at a ratio of 1 teaspoon of oil per 4 cups (1 L) of water, and use the entire mixture at once. (Otherwise, the oil will settle; it does not emulsify well.) Keep agitating the container as you use it. Though not always necessary, you can add a wetting agent, such as yucca (see page 105) or a few drops of nonphosphate soap, which helps the spray adhere to the leaf. Make sure the neem oil is from an organic source and of high quality. Only use during vegetative growth. To limit the possibility of neem oil reacting with the sun and burning the leaves of your plant, only spray late in the day or around sunset.

>>>>> Natural Insecticide Spray

You can use this base recipe to make a number of insecticidal sprays with plants that have natural insecticidal properties. You can use plants that you may already have growing in your garden or ones that you would like to plant in the coming seasons, depending on what you have available to you.

What You Need

2 cups (480 ml) water

1 handful fresh plant matter (see list in the next column for options) or 50–75 drops (½–¾ teaspoons) rosemary, thyme, oregano, or eucalyptus essential oils

1. Heat the water to a boil. Combine the plants with the hot water and let steep with the lid on for 2 hours. If you're using essential oils, let the water cool before adding essential oils or add them right before use.

2. Strain the mixture into a spray bottle. Compost the plant material. To apply, spray the mixture directly on the insects or their eggs.

Tip: Always be conscious that there are other beneficial insects in your garden that you want to encourage and keep healthy. Try your best to avoid spraying any beneficial insects.

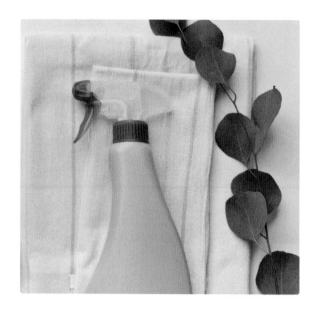

PLANTS FOR NATURAL INSECTICIDE SPRAY

Cayenne peppers (chopped)

Chrysanthemum flower

Cloves (crushed with a mortar and pestle or chopped)

Garlic cloves (diced)

Jerusalem artichoke

Lemon balm

Mugwort

Pine, spruce, fir, and hemlock needles

Rosemary

Stinging nettle

Tansy

Thyme

Tobacco leaves (fresh or dried, broken up into small pieces)

Wormwood

Yarrow

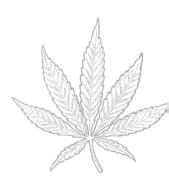

BENEFICIAL INSECTS (AND OTHER HELPFUL ORGANISMS)

Beneficial insects can be purchased through various insectaries throughout North America (and beyond). For some growers, it can be even more effective to cultivate plants that can provide a habitat for these insects alongside your cannabis. The ability to identify and understand the breeding, biology, and behavior of these insects and their host plants is another amazing tool to have at your disposal.

Aphidius colemani: This parasitic wasp preys on the green peach aphid (*Myzus persicae*) and the melon aphid (*Aphis gossypii*), which is also known as the cotton aphid.

Dicyphus hesperus: This predator feeds on whiteflies, thrips, aphids, moth eggs, and other pests. Be careful for it does feed on plant tissue as well.

Green lacewing (*Chrysoperla rufilabris*): The predatory larva of the green lacewing feeds on aphids.

Ground beetles (*Carabidae* family): The term *ground beetles* commonly refers to over two thousand species of nocturnal beetles in North America. They consume slugs and snails, mites, caterpillars, earwigs, cutworms, vine borers, aphids, and lots of other insects. Most are dark and shiny, with ridged wing covers. Consider building a beetle bank to provide a habitat for these beneficial midnight marauders!

Hoverflies (*Syrphidae* family): Also called flower flies or syrphid flies, hoverflies feed mainly on nectar and pollen as adults, but the larvae feed voraciously on aphids, thrips, and other plant-sucking insects.

Insidious flower bug (*Orius insidiosus*): This minute pirate bug feeds on adult thrips, aphids, small caterpillars, mites, and the eggs of various small insects.

Ladybugs (*Coccinellidae family*): There are many species of ladybugs that feed on pests such as aphids and scale.

Neoseiulus californicus: This predatory mite will feed on the two-spotted spider mite.

Parasitoid wasps (*Hymenoptera order*): There are a number of small parasitic wasps that will lay their eggs in many cannabis plant pests, including aphids.

Steinernema feltiae: This nematode lives in the soil and feeds on many different pests, including fungus gnats and thrips.

Stratiolaelaps scimitus: Formerly *Hypoaspis miles*, this mite species lives in soil and feeds on fungus gnats.

COMMON PESTS

This section will cover the most common pests that are found on cannabis and some options for controlling infestations, including descriptions of store-bought products, a list of beneficial organisms, and suggestions for homemade treatments. Different pests may be present in your specific area. If you're interested in learning more, it might be helpful to pick up another book or two (see "Resources," page 233) that goes into much more detail than we are able to cover in this one chapter.

Many of these pests are more detrimental to indoor plants. They can also be a problem for outdoor plants, but there are more chances that beneficial organisms may come to your rescue.

Fungus Gnats

Fungus gnats can do considerable damage to the root zone of indoor plants if left unchecked.

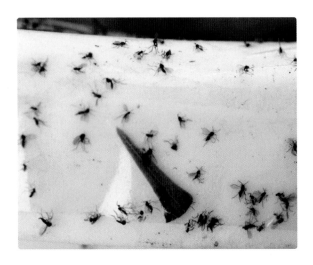

These small black flies lay their eggs in the top layer of soil and thrive in moist, soggy, over-watered pots. The larvae that hatch from the eggs feed on roots, leaving them susceptible to other diseases and fungal infections. You will discover their presence if you see the adult flies hovering over your soil.

Pest Control Options

Beneficial organisms: *Steinernema feltiae* (see page 207), *Stratiolaelaps scimitus* (see page 207).

Helpful products: Apply a microbial insecticide containing *Bacillus thuringiensis* (BT), a naturally occurring soil-borne bacterium that can fight fungus gnats and other pests.

Homemade treatments: Let the top layer of your pots dry out between waterings. Place yellow sticky traps near the soil to catch the adult flies and make you aware of their presence.

You can add 50 drops each (1 teaspoon) of rosemary and clove essential oils (or 100 drops or 2 teaspoons of just one of these oils) to 4 cups (1 L) of cold water. To use fresh or dried rosemary and cloves instead, add one cup of each plant (or 2 cups of one of the plants) to 8 cups (2 L) of hot water. Let the tea steep overnight, then strain. Either spray the essential oil mixture or the tea onto the top layer of your soil or use it to lightly water the top layer of your soil for two consecutive waterings. Reapply if needed.

Two-Spotted Spider Mites

These mites can be found on the undersides of leaves. They thrive and will breed quickly in hot and dry conditions (85°F–90°F [29°C–32°C] and 50 percent humidity). Look out for tiny pinpricks or dots of yellow on the top side of the leaves. If you see little webs on the underside of the leaves, this means that the mites have been living on your plants for a while and are most likely well-established.

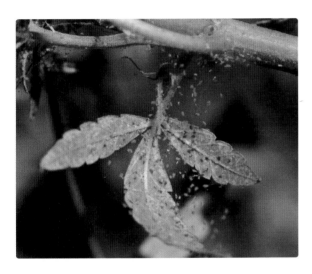

Pest Control Options

Beneficial organisms: Predatory mites, such as *Phytoseiulus persimilis*, *Neoseiulus californicus*, and *Amblyseius andersoni*.

Helpful products: Apply insecticidal soap, natural oil–based sprays (see page 206), or neem-based oils on the leaves. A foliar spray (see page 68) made from kelp extract can also be helpful for killing spider-mite eggs.

Homemade treatments: Wash your plants with a wet cloth and a bucket of water, making sure to rub the undersides of each leaf and then rinse the cloth in the bucket of warm water. It is tedious and painstaking work, but physically removing the spider mites will allow you to knock down their population and then take another action to control them.

Thrips

Thrips are small, cylindrical-shaped insects that are off-white or brown in color. The adults are capable of growing wings. You will find them mainly on the underside of leaves. They have a rasplike mouth that they use to suck out the fluid from the leaves. This causes them to lose chlorophyll and leaves behind small, silver blotches.

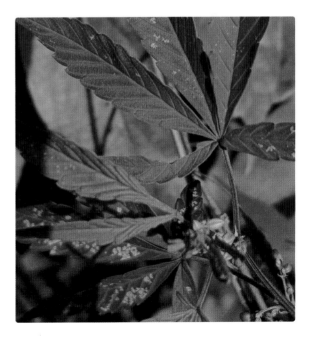

Pest Control Options

Beneficial organisms: *Neoseiulus cucumeris* (a predatory mite that feeds on the thrip nymph), *Orius insidiosus* (a minute pirate bug that feeds on adult thrips), *Steinernema feltiae* (see page 207), *Stratiolaelaps scimitus* (see page 207), and *Amblyseius swirskii* (a predatory mite).

Helpful products: Apply insecticidal soap or neem oil to the leaves. *Beauveria bassiana* is a fungus (a microbial insecticide), which causes a disease known as the white muscadine disease in insects.

Homemade treatments: Place yellow sticky strips around the plant to catch the thrips.

Broad Mites and Hemp Russet Mites

These mites suck the juices out of the plant stems and leaves. They are only 0.5 millimeter in size and are hard to see with the naked eye, but if leaves begin to droop and curl and often have a glossy or wet appearance, these mites may be feeding on your plants.

Pest Control Options

Beneficial organisms: *Neoseiulus californicus* (a predatory mite) and *Amblyseius andersoni* (a predatory mite that is effective at both cold and high temperatures).

Helpful products: Apply insecticidal soap, natural oil–based sprays, or neem oil to the leaves.

Homemade treatments: Use trap plants (see page 202), such as broad beans, to draw these mites away from your cannabis plants.

Aphids and Cannabis Aphids

There are a number of different aphid species that can be found on cannabis (peach, cotton, and potato, to name a few). The cannabis aphid is becoming very prevalent in North America and is proving to be a formidable foe. This pest can feed on sap from the plant's leaves and stems and will reproduce heavily on outdoor grown cannabis. (Aphids are often more common in outdoor gardens than indoor gardens.) Aphids will often excrete a liquid substance called honeydew that can attract ants and create potential issues with mold.

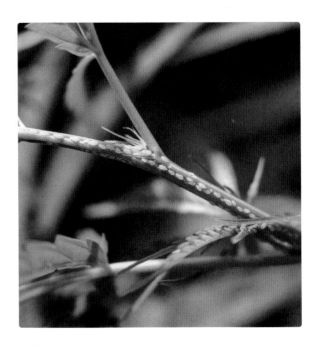

Pest Control Options

Beneficial organisms: Green lacewing (see page 207), ladybugs (page 207), *Aphidoletes aphidimyza* (a predatory midge that feeds on many species of aphids), and parasitic wasps, including *Aphidius colemani* (see page 207), *Aphidius ervi* (attacks many species of larger aphids), *Aphidius matricariae* (can control almost forty species of aphids), and *Aphelinus abdominalis* (feeds on aphid nymphs).

Helpful products: Apply insecticidal soap, natural oil–based sprays (see page 206), or neem oil to the leaves. You can also use a microbial spray with *Beauveria bassiana*.

Homemade treatments: Create a homemade alcohol and water solution by combining 2 cups (470 ml) water, 2 cups 70 percent isopropyl alcohol (or 1½ cups [375 ml] water and 1 cup [240 ml] 90 percent isopropyl alcohol). You can add a tablespoon (15 ml) of insecticidal soap to this mixture to increase its effectiveness. Spray the leaves of your plant with this solution every 3–4 days. You can also blast the aphids with water from a hose and make them fall to the ground. It will not kill the bugs by any means, but it will knock them back and slow the infestation.

Whiteflies

These flies resemble tiny, white moths. The adults lay their eggs on the undersides of the leaves. The larvae will feed on the leaves and create a shiny coating on the topside. Eventually, the leaves will yellow, and you will notice the overall health of the affected plant decline.

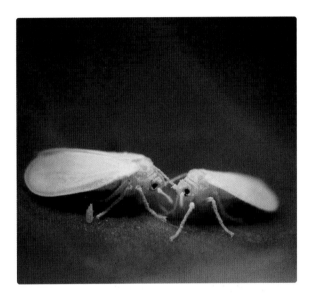

Pest Control Options

Beneficial organisms: *Amblyseius swirskii* (a predatory mite), *Dicyphus hesperus* (see page 207), and *Delphastus catalinae* (a member of the ladybird beetle family that preys on whiteflies, also called the whitefly lady beetle).

Helpful products: Apply insecticidal soap, natural oil–based sprays (see page 206), or neem oil to the leaves. You can also use a microbial insecticide with *Beauveria bassiana*.

Homemade treatments: You can use the natural insecticidal soap recipe on page 206 to treat a whitefly infestation.

Slugs and Snails

Slugs and snails can be a problem, especially with younger plants and seedlings. They will feed on the tissue of your plants and, in some cases, consume entire seedlings. In older plants, they can weaken the stems and feed on the leaves. You will notice their slimy trails on your plants.

Pest Control Options

Beneficials: Ground beetles (both adults and larva, see page 207) and leopard slugs (feeds on other slugs).

Helpful products: There are some pelleted slug deterrents on the market that contain iron phosphate and will kill slugs.

Homemade treatments: You can make a simple vinegar spray that can kill slugs or snails. Mix 2 parts vinegar to 1 part water and spray on any that you see.

To prevent them from reaching your plants, cover your seedling trays with humidity domes. Wool can work as a deterrent if you spread it around the base of your plants. You can also spread a barrier of diatomaceous earth around the perimeter of your plants. Slugs and snails do not like to crawl across it.

To draw snails and slugs away from your plants, create a beer or yeast trap. Put a little beer or yeast and water in shallow containers and place them on the edges of your gardens. The slugs and snails will be attracted to these areas.

Mammals

Generally speaking, cannabis is most susceptible to various mammals when in the seedling or the beginning of the vegetative stage. For example, mice and voles will dig up plants, eat seeds, and chew down small seedlings. Mammals pose more of a problem in the spring, when your plants are small and there is not a lot of lush green growth on the landscape. Once a plant has grown to about 2 feet (61 cm), it tends to repel most herbivores with its natural defense systems. If you have ever eaten a cannabis leaf, you will know full well that it does not taste good.

I have mostly only had issues with animals such as deer, rabbits, and porcupines feeding on smaller plants, though one year a porcupine chewed down and ate the vast majority of an 8-foot (2.4-m) tall plant. I'm sure he was feeling it as he wandered away into the forest.

Homemade treatments: If you are worried, you can try fencing off or covering your plants with a cage when they are young. You can keep young plants in containers away from the ground on tables and wrap aluminum foil (or a similarly smooth material) around the legs of the table to prevent small mammals from climbing up them.

Another preventive measure for both large and small animals is to provide an alternative food source to lure them away from your plants. This could mean planting lettuce or other lush greens for rabbits, deer, and groundhogs around the perimeter of your garden. Each location and bioregion will be different, and to use this tactic, it is important for you to understand the food choices, biology, and behavior of your local wildlife.

COMMON DISEASES

Diseases, especially those caused by fungi or mold, can wreak havoc on cannabis. At some point, you are going to encounter at least one of these conditions. This section will give you some tips and ideas on how to deal with them.

Powdery Mildew

Powdery mildew (PM for short) thrives in humid conditions and when there is a large fluctuation in daytime and nighttime temperatures. This fungal issue can affect both indoor and outdoor growers, and can quickly get out of control and ruin your crop. The mildew looks like a dusty-white substance that first appears on the leaves and can quickly spread to the entire plant, including the buds. From there, it can travel throughout your garden, with devastating results.

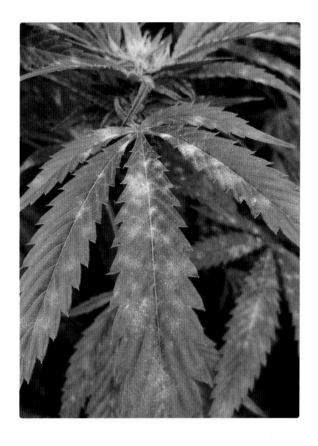

Treatment Options

Helpful products: Neem oil can disrupt the metabolism of PM and stop spore production. It can be used both as a treatment and a preventive measure. Mix 3 tablespoons (45 ml) per 1 gallon (3.8 L) of warm water and shake vigorously before applying to the leaves. It can be used every 7–10 days during vegetative growth. Do not use when the plants have begun flowering.

Homemade treatments: You can make a wide range of sprays at home. Potassium bicarbonate changes the pH of the surface of the leaf, creating an unsuitable environment for PM to grow. Add 3 tablespoons (45 ml) of potassium bicarbonate, 3 tablespoons (45 ml) of vegetable oil, and 1¼ teaspoons (6 ml) of natural dish soap into 1 gallon (3.8 L) of water. Mix together and apply the spray onto the leaves every 4–7 days until the mildew subsides.

For mild cases or as a preventive, baking soda can be effective. Like potassium carbonate, it has a very high pH and creates an alkaline environment that can kill the fungus. Mix 1 tablespoon (15 ml) of baking soda, 1–2 teaspoons (5–10 ml) of natural dish soap, and 1 gallon (3.8 L) of water. Spray at the end of the day when the sun is setting to avoid sunburn. It can be reapplied once a week when used as a preventive measure.

You can also try making a simple spray by mixing milk and water, using a ratio of 1 part milk to 2 parts water or combining 1 ounce (28 g) of powdered milk with a half gallon (2 L) of water. The milk acts as a natural fungicide and boosts the plant's natural immune system.

The acetic acid in apple cider vinegar will help treat mild cases of PM. Mix 4 tablespoons (60 ml) of vinegar and 1 gallon (3.8 L) of water. Make sure you do not make the solution too strong, as vinegar can burn the plants. Reapply every 3 days or so. Spray at the end of the day when the sun is setting to avoid sunburn.

Prevention: Powdery mildew thrives in moist, humid conditions. Maintaining a dry and stable humidity level under 45 percent can go a long way if PM is a problem for you. Although this is under the recommended humidity level for optimal growth, it will help to prevent and limit its spread. Avoid crowding your plants and make sure to have adequate airflow around and through the branches, increasing air circulation and ventilation if needed. If possible, isolate any plants that start to show signs of PM before it infects others.

It is also best to try to keep the temperature as stable as possible. Changes in temperature of more than 9°F (5°C) from the day to the night cycle will increase the chances of fungal spores settling with the dew that forms on your plants. Do not spray water on your plants and let them sit all night long when they are wet. Instead, use any sprays and water in the morning and then let plants dry throughout the day. You may also want to allow your growing medium to dry out a bit between waterings so that it does not remain wet and soggy for long periods of time.

Spraying your plants with aerated compost tea (as outlined on page 136) will prevent PM from forming and benefit your plant nutritionally as well. The microbes in the tea will take up the space that the mildew would need to grow and protect against its spores.

When possible, look for cultivars that are PM-resistant.

Botrytis

Botrytis is one of the most common fungal issues that cannabis growers will face, attacking your buds and ruining your flowers. It begins forming on the stem and inside your buds. In wet conditions, it will quickly spread throughout the bud. In seedlings, it can result in damping off. Damping off is a disease that affects the stem and roots of the plant. The stem near the soil surface will begin to rot and become mushy as the plant wilts, falls over, and dies.

It can be hard for the untrained eye to spot this fungal enemy until it is too late. Botrytis can vary from greenish-blue to white-gray. It tends to wreak the most havoc on plants that have tight, dense buds. If found, cut out the affected plant material right away and discard it. The spores can become airborne, so be careful when moving an affected plant around and always sterilize the tools you use.

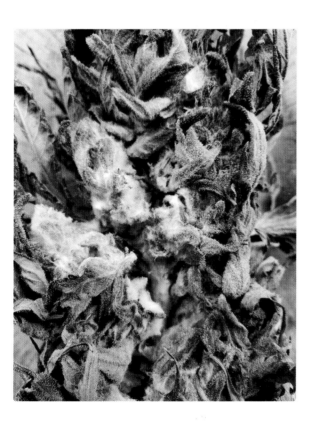

Treatment Options

Products: Using a spray with *Bacillus subtilis* can be a good preventive method, but if your plants are in flower, I do not recommend spraying anything. Sometimes, you need to cut your losses.

Prevention: Be sure to closely inspect your buds, paying close attention to the areas around the stalks at the center of the bud. Harvest your plants before the cold, wet rains of fall begin. Make sure there is good airflow around your plants and try to maintain a humidity around 50 percent. Also look for cultivars that are mold-resistant and thrive in wet and humid conditions if you live in this type of environment. Discard any material that has gray mold. Do not try to save anything that has been infected—it is not worth it.

Some herbs such as chamomile, cinnamon, and garlic have antifungal properties and can be brewed into a plant tea (see the recipe on page 133) or a foliar spray that you can apply to your cannabis as a preventive measure.

Pythium

Pythium is a fungus that can cause damping off in seedlings and clones. It uses decaying root matter to spread and causes healthy roots to die. Plants with pythium will experience a reduction in nutrient and water uptake, a yellowing of the plant tissues, and a slowdown in growth. Once your plant has pythium, it will always have it, and it can pass it to any cuttings. You can manage pythium, but the health of the plant will be forever compromised.

Treatment Options

Helpful products: Use bacterial enzymes, available in bottled form that can be mixed with water, to help break down dead and decaying root matter. Bacteria such as *Bacillus subtilis* can be helpful in limiting the effects of this disease.

Homemade treatments: You can make horsetail tea using the recipe on page 133 and use it for watering. Horsetail is a natural fungicide. Water and use a foliar spray with compost teas (especially ones rich in beneficial bacteria and mycorrhizae).

Prevention: Maintaining a dry and stable humidity level of 45 percent stops pythium from spreading throughout your crop. Let your soil dry out between waterings. Provide and maintain a soil that has a healthy balance of microbes and fungal life.

You also want to maintain and support a healthy balance of microbes, bacteria, and mycorrhizae in your soil. Doing so will protect against this and many other conditions. Make sure your water is at or just below 65°F (18.5°C) and keep your water well-oxygenated using an air pump.

Fusarium

Fusarium is a fungus that causes a form of leaf blight. It begins in the soil. The base of your plant then turns brown, and the aboveground parts of the plant will yellow and wilt, as the disease progresses and the roots of the plant rot.

Treatment Options

Helpful products: A foliar spray with sulfur can work as a fungicide (and insecticide), but it should be used as a last resort. Do not mix sulfur sprays and horticultural oils or neem oil, and wait at least a week between treatments using these products. Fungi such as *Trichoderma* spp. and bacteria such as *Bacillus subtilis* can be helpful in limiting the effects of this disease.

Homemade treatments: Water and foliar spray with compost teas (especially ones rich in beneficial bacteria and mycorrhizae) and keep your growing area as clean as possible. You can also heat the soil to kill the fungal spores by covering the infected area with a black tarp.

Other: As with all fungal diseases, maintain a dry and stable humidity level of 45 percent, allow your growing medium to dry out a bit between waterings, and increase your air circulation and ventilation. Always work with clean and sterile tools, as fungal infections can easily be spread through contaminated tools. If fusarium is found in your outdoor soil, do not plant next year's plants in the same location.

whereas indoor plants are often forced to work with whatever nutrients are available from a formulated, liquid solution.

Nutrient deficiencies are more common than excesses. In most cases, a plant will not absorb a nutrient that it does not need, even if it's available in the soil. But if a nutrient is lacking, the plant does not have any other means to find it and will therefore suffer.

NUTRIENT IMBALANCES

When plants do not have access to all the nutrients that they need or have more nutrients than they can absorb, they will begin to show signs that something is wrong. For any nutrient imbalance, it will be up to you to step up and deliver what your plant seeks. The descriptions of nutrient balances in this section will help you to build your knowledge and experience, listen to your intuition, and hone your gardening sixth sense.

These deficiencies and excesses are less common in outdoor plants growing in living soil than in plants grown indoors using a soilless medium and bottled nutrients. Plants in living soil will seek out and absorb the nutrients that they need at any given time,

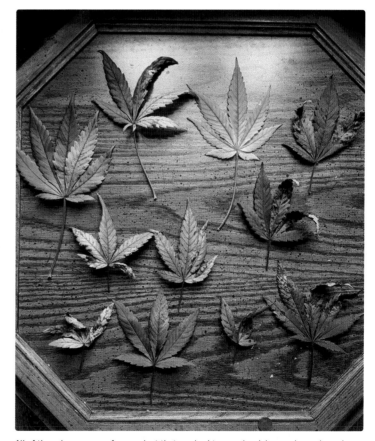

All of these leaves came from a plant that received too much calcium and experienced nutrient lockout as a result. These leaves show signs of several deficiencies, including those of nitrogen, potassium, and iron.

As with pests, it is best to use preventive measures when it comes to nutrient deficiencies and excesses in your soil. When using high-quality living soil, whether you purchase it from a reputable source, mix up your own, or supplement your native living soil with amendments, make sure that the plant has everything it needs readily available from the start. This way, you do not have to figure out what to add and how to add it later.

Like everything else about plant care, it can take time to be able to properly and accurately diagnose a nutrient imbalance. Sometimes, the symptoms are blatantly obvious, but in other instances, they come in the form of subtle color changes. Again, simple observation and awareness will go a long way toward keeping your plants thriving and healthy.

If your plants are suffering from a deficiency, look to pages 71–77 to learn about soil amendments that can provide the missing nutrients. Flushing your soil with water can combat nutrient excesses, but, again, with healthy, living soils, these excesses are rarely a problem. Another point for living soils!

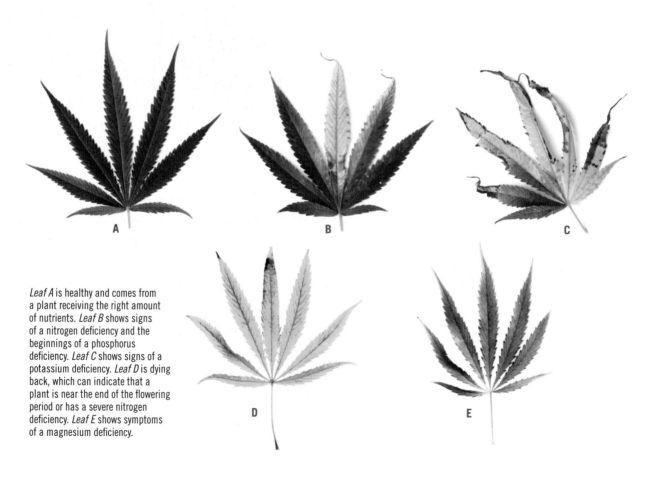

Leaf A is healthy and comes from a plant receiving the right amount of nutrients. *Leaf B* shows signs of a nitrogen deficiency and the beginnings of a phosphorus deficiency. *Leaf C* shows signs of a potassium deficiency. *Leaf D* is dying back, which can indicate that a plant is near the end of the flowering period or has a severe nitrogen deficiency. *Leaf E* shows symptoms of a magnesium deficiency.

Nitrogen

Nitrogen is a key nutrient for growth. If there is a nitrogen deficiency, older leaves will start to yellow as the plant allocates resources from existing growth to support new growth. If left unchecked, the yellowing will gradually move up the plant. Older leaves will turn brown, shrivel up, and fall off the plant. You will also notice decreased growth; sometimes, growth might stall altogether.

If there is excess nitrogen, the leaves of the plant will turn a very dark, dull, and deep green color. Vegetative growth may be prolonged and last long into the flowering cycle. The leaves may curl under, and the branches and stalks may become brittle and easily breakable.

Phosphorus

Phosphorus helps your plants convert and utilize other nutrients in your soil. It is also very important for the flowering stage. When a plant is deficient in phosphorus, the leaf tips will darken and curl upward, and the leaves and leaf stems may take on a purple appearance. Dark blotches will develop on the leaves, and growth will slow.

When a plant has too much phosphorus, it can start to lock out other nutrients, such as calcium, magnesium, zinc, and iron. You may notice white coloring between the veins and yellowing of the leaves. Phosphorus excess can be tricky to diagnose, as this yellowing is often a sign of many other nutrient deficiencies.

Potassium

Potassium helps transport water throughout the entire plant. It is also used in photosynthesis and helps to control the opening and closing of the stomata. When lacking in potassium, the leaf tips and edges will appear burned, and the leaves may develop spots before curling up and falling off the plant.

The signs of potassium excess are very similar to those of an excess of phosphorus. Look for a light yellow or whitish color between the leaf veins.

Calcium

Calcium helps plants to build healthy and strong cell walls and absorb potassium. When plants are not receiving enough calcium, they will snap and break easily, and the leaves will display yellow or rust-colored patches that will continue to spread.

Calcium excess leads to the lockout of various nutrients, such as potassium, magnesium, manganese, and iron. It is important to note that having too much calcium in your soil may be causing other nutrient deficiencies in your plants. In other words, if you are seeing signs of deficiencies in your plants, be aware that too much calcium may be the cause.

Magnesium

Magnesium is needed in order for the plant to metabolize phosphorus and to produce chlorophyll, which in turn allows your plant to use sunlight for photosynthesis. A magnesium deficiency is one of the most common nutrient-related issues affecting cannabis plants. It will lead to yellowing that starts on the lower branches of a plant and moves toward the top of the plant, if it is not corrected.

Although rare, excess magnesium will inhibit the absorption of calcium and result in stunted growth and weak plants.

Sulfur

Sulfur is needed for chlorophyll production. If your plants have a sulfur deficiency, you will see yellowing on new growth, and the overall plant growth will slow down and may become stunted if the deficiency is serious. If your plants are low in sulfur they will most likely be low in nitrogen as well.

Excess sulfur will make soil more acidic and slow the growth of your plants. In most cases, being careful when adding any kind of sulfur to your soil and addressing a potential nitrogen imbalance will take care of this condition. Sulfur deficiencies are very uncommon and experienced very rarely by growers.

Iron

Plants use iron for a number of metabolic functions, including chlorophyll production and nitrogen fixation. Iron deficiencies are fairly common in plants that are not grown in a healthy, living soil. It often presents itself first in the yellowing of new growth and the upper leaves. The leaf tips will turn yellow while the leaf veins remain green.

Too much iron in your soil interferes with the plant's ability to make and maintain healthy chlorophyll, causing the leaves of affected plants to develop bronze speckling.

FAQS & TROUBLESHOOTING

Q: Is there a surefire way to tell exactly what nutrient deficiency is affecting my plants?

A: You can send your leaf tissue samples to a lab to be diagnosed, but this is not an option for everyone. Without testing, the information contained in this chapter and in other resources can serve as guideposts. Different nutrient deficiencies often present themselves in similar ways so they can be tricky to diagnose. Just do your best, and as you try different remedies and options, you will in time become better at identifying and rectifying these issues as they arise.

Q: What should I do if I notice mold on my buds?

A: It is not good to have mold of any kind on your buds, but, fortunately, you do not need to throw out your entire plant. Instead, cut the infected area out and discard them far away from your garden. Don't try to save or salvage anything that is moldy. Cut and discard above and below the infected area as well. Keep a close eye for any more mold that may appear and continue to get rid of the affected parts as they pop up. If mold continues to be an issue, it is best to harvest your plants, cut out any infected areas, and get your plants drying as soon as possible. Be sure to clean and sterilize your scissors or cutting device afterwards with alcohol to avoid spreading the mold.

Q: If I use a treatment and it stops being effective on a specific pest, what should I do?

A: Simply switch to another product. When using any natural biological treatments (whether you're using store-bought or homemade ones), it can be a good idea to switch between products anyway so that the pests do not adapt to your treatments.

Q: Should I try new products at full strength?

A: When using a new product or treatment (even a homemade one), always test it out on one plant first and at half strength. Take time to see how that plant reacts before applying it to your entire garden. This advice applies when you're treating a pest or a disease as well as when applying nutrients or fertilizer. It is a simple step that could save you from damaging or destroying an entire crop.

Q: Can I spray my plants during the flowering stage?

A: No, *never* spray anything on your plants when they are flowering. It is better to lose a plant or two (or even an entire crop) than to risk contaminating your harvest. I avoid spraying anything (even natural sprays or pure water) during the flowering stage.

< GLOSSARY >

autoflower Variety of cannabis that is not photoperiod-dependent. It will automatically enter the flowering stage after a given period of time, rather than in response to decreasing amounts of daylight.

bioavailable A term describing nutrients or other substances that are in a form that can be absorbed by the plant and distributed throughout its vascular system.

biological controls Living organisms that are the natural enemies of pests and control pest populations. These include beneficial insects, such as mites, and microorganisms, such as soil fungi and bacteria.

biomass The organic matter that is produced by the plants in your garden during each growing season. Biomass should be left to decompose in your garden beds or compost pile so the nutrients it contains return to your soil.

biostimulant A microorganism or substance used to help your cannabis plants absorb nutrients, adapt to stress, or increase quality or yield. They support the health of your plants and can be very effective.

bottled nutrients A mixture of nutrients and water that are bottled and sold commercially.

buds The clusters of flowers that are often covered in resin or trichomes. This part of the plant contains the precious cannabinoids, terpenes, flavonoids, and other chemical constituents of cannabis. They are also referred to as nugs, nuggets, or "colas."

burping The process of opening the containers that your cannabis is curing in to release stale air and moisture, and allow new air to come in. This is often done when people are curing cannabis in glass jars or rubber totes.

calyx Another word for the sepals of a plant, which protect the plant's flower and reproductive organs.

cannabinoids Chemical compounds found in cannabis. There are more than a hundred different cannabinoids. The best-known ones include THC, CBD, CBC, and CBG.

CBD (cannabidiol) A major nonpsychoactive cannabinoid that is found in highest concentrations in the flowers or buds of the cannabis plant. It has many medicinal properties and can be taken internally in various forms, such as through smoking, vaping, edibles, and tinctures.

chemovar Categories used to classify varieties of cannabis, based on their chemical makeup. Scientists look at the presence and quantity of various cannabinoids, terpenes, and other constituents, such as lipids and waxes, to determine the differences between chemovars.

clone	A cutting that is a genetic copy of the parent plant it was taken from. Many growers propagate cannabis through cloning, taking one or more cuttings from a desirable female mother plant.
closed-loop system	In farming, a closed-loop system mimics nature and offers a way to harness and recycle energy and nutrients back into your farm (or garden) without relying on outside inputs, and disperse it in a way that adds to the health and vitality of your local environment.
cola	The large cluster of flowers (see "buds") located on the top of the branches of a cannabis plant.
compost	Decomposed organic matter that is used to deliver nutrients to your plants and help to condition or improve the health of your soil.
cultivar	This term is short for "cultivated variety." Distinct cultivars are made by selecting and breeding for specific traits that are deemed desirable, such as potency, smell, plant structure, and the like. Many people refer to cultivars as "strains" in the cannabis community. I prefer to use the term "cultivar."
curing	A slow drying process that allows flowers to retain much of their smell and terpenes and will make them taste and burn better and more consistently. Most growers will cure their flowers for 1–2 months.
damping off	A fungal disease that affects the stem and roots of the plant and causes its stem to rot. An affected plant will wilt and eventually fall over and die.
dioecious	Referring to plants in which the female and male flowers grow on separate plants.
dry trim	A type of trimming that involves removing all the leaves from the flowers after the plant is fully dried. This can be done just before or just after the curing process. Most growers agree that dry trimming will produce a final product with superior taste, smell, and potency.
endocannabinoid system (ECS)	
	A signaling system in the body that maintains homeostasis. It regulates immune response, emotions, motor function, inflammation, blood pressure, appetite, memory, bone growth, pain, decision-making, and more. The ECS consists of receptors spread throughout the tissues within the body that react to endocannabinoids (which are produced by our body) and phytocannabinoids (which are produced by cannabis and some other plants).
evaporation	The process by which water turns from liquid to water vapor. Most of the water that moves through a plant's vascular system is lost to evaporation.
fan leaves	Large, primary leaves that contain anywhere from three to nine leaflets. They are full of flavonoids, vitamins, and minerals, and are often used for juicing but not for smoking. They have become a symbol that is known around the world and associated with the cannabis plant.

feminized seeds Seeds that have been bred so as to produce only female plants. They are generally produced through a process of stressing a female plant to the point that it produces male flowers that pollinate the female flowers on the plant.

fimming A pruning technique in which growers take off part of the main growing shoot; this increases lateral branching and the number of growing shoots and flowering sites.

foliar feeding The act of delivering nutrients to your plants by mixing the nutrients with water and spraying the solution onto your plants. It is a very quick and efficient way to deliver nutrients to your plants, especially if they are experiencing a nutrient deficiency.

fungicide A chemical or biological organism that is used to eradicate fungal diseases.

genotype The set of genes that a living organism has, including genes that determine traits such as the height of the plant, the color of its pistils, or its disease resistance.

hermaphrodite A term used to describe cannabis plants that contain both male and female flowers on the same plant. Hermaphrodites are undesirable and will pass this trait on to future offspring.

high-stress training

A collection of training techniques that involve removing parts of the plant and/or injuring the plant to optimize growth and increase yield. It is more invasive than low-stress training.

inflorescence A grouping of flowers at the top of the stem or another main branch of a plant. The inflorescence of cannabis is referred to as the "cola."

integrated pest management (IPM) protocol

A series of principles and practices that allow you to survey, detect, and address any pest or disease ssues in your garden.

kief The product that results from sifting or rubbing your dried flowers or sugar leaves through a sieve or screen to separate the trichomes or resin heads from the buds. A form of dry sift hash, it is one of the easiest and simplest extractions you can do at home.

larf The small and undesirable buds located near the bottom of your plants. Once dried, they are very small and of limited value. These small flowers are also referred to as "minging buds."

leaf axis The place where the petiole meets the stem of a plant.

light deprivation A technique of inducing a cannabis plant to go into flower earlier than it naturally would by decreasing the amount of light that the plant receives. Most growers will pull tarps over hoops or use some kind of "blackout" cloth that decreases the amount of light that the plants receive to 12 hours over a 24-hour period.

living soil

Soil that contains organic material and is alive with a diverse mix of living organisms, including bacteria, fungi, protozoa, worms, nematodes, yeasts, and algae. These organisms work together to break down organic material and deliver nutrients to the roots of your plants.

low-stress training

A collection of training practices that increase yields, encourage horizontal growth, and increase the number of flower sites with minimal impact to the plant. It is generally done when your plants are young and includes techniques such as bending and tying your plants.

manure

Animal waste or feces that are broken down and decomposed, and then added to the soil to deliver nutrients that help your plants grow and thrive.

microbial pesticide

Natural organisms, such as fungi, viruses, bacteria, and protozoa, that are used to combat pests or diseases. They are much less toxic than chemical pesticides.

mycorrhizae

Fungi that grow symbiotically with the roots of plants. In Latin, *myco* means "fungi" and *rhiza* means "root."

petiole

The stalk of the leaf that attaches the leaf to the stem of the plant.

pH

A measure of the acidity or alkalinity of a substance. Seven is considered neutral; anything below this measurement is considered acidic and anything above this number is considered alkaline.

phenotype

The observable physical characteristics that are a result of an organism's genes and environmental factors. Examples of a plant's phenotype include the color and shape of the leaves, the structure of growth, and the density of trichomes.

photoperiod-dependent

A term to describe plants that begin the flowering stage based on the amount of available daylight over a 24-hour period.

pinching

A pruning technique that encourages the plant to produce two main growing shoots instead of one. It is done by cutting or "pinching" the top of the plant to encourage two new shoots to grow from the leaf axis of the plant. It can be done over and over again, resulting in a shorter, bushier plant with many main growing shoots.

polyculture gardening

Growing many different species of plants in a garden to increase the biodiversity of the area. Unlike monoculture gardening, which involves cultivating a single species, polyculture gardening is much more sustainable, supports much more life in your garden, and brings many benefits to your cannabis plants.

ppm (parts per million)

A unit of measurement to describe the total dissolved solids (see "total dissolved solids") in your water. Whereas 1 percent would be 1 part of 100, this measurement would be 1 part of 10,000.

regenerative farming

A group of farming principles and practices that encourage biodiversity and help to regenerate and enhance the health of a farm, its soil, and the ecosystem as a whole.

regular seeds   Seeds that have an equal chance of sprouting into a male or a female plant.

sinsemilla   Based on the Spanish words for "without seeds" (*sin semilla*), this refers to flowers that remain unpollinated. If unpollinated, the flowers will continue to grow bigger and produce more resin, resulting in larger buds that are more potent.

soil amendment   A substance that is added to your garden to increase the physical or chemical quality of the soil.

soilless   A term describing substances used to grow cannabis that do not contain living organisms, such as peat moss, rockwool, clay pellets, and perlite. It is a medium that does not contain soil. Many soilless potting mixes contain peat and perlite, and are considered sterile, so as to limit the growth of unwanted bacteria or fungi that could potentially lead to disease.

stacking function   A principle within "regenerative farming" that revolves around having every aspect or element in your garden serve multiple purposes. It allows you to maximize output with the least amount of input.

stomata   The tiny pores located on the leaves and stems of plants that take in carbon dioxide and release oxygen into the air.

strain   See "cultivar."

sugar leaves   Small leaves that are located around and interspersed with cannabis flowers. They are covered in trichomes and can be used to make various products, such as edibles, salves, and tinctures.

sweating   The act of laying out your cannabis on screens or a table to allow the excess moisture to evaporate during the curing process (after they have been sealed in a container, jar, or tote). If your buds are too wet, you will need to remove some excess moisture to achieve a proper cure.

terpenes   Organic compounds that are mainly found in the essential oils and resins of many plants and trees. Terpenes are responsible for the distinctive taste and aroma of the many different cultivars of cannabis.

THC (tetrahydrocannabinol)

The principal psychoactive cannabinoid that is found in highest concentrations in the flowers or buds of the cannabis plant. It has many medicinal properties and can be taken internally through various forms, such as smoking, vaping, edibles, and tinctures.

top-dress   To spread something, such as a soil amendment, on top of the soil.

total dissolved solids (TDS)

The concentration of organic and inorganic substances found in your water or soil. It is often measured in parts per million (see "ppm"). You can purchase a TDS meter to take this measurement.

transpiration   The process of water moving through a plant and its evaporation from the stems, leaves, and flowers. Plants use very little of the water that moves through their vascular tissue, sometimes as little as 0.5 percent.

trichomes   Found on cannabis flowers and some leaves, trichomes are substances that act as a natural defense for the plants, protecting them from animals and the sun. These trichomes are very resinous and contain the sought-after cannabinoids and terpenes that have made cannabis such an important plant around the world.

trim containers   Two nested containers, one with a screen in the bottom to separate trichomes from the rest of the plant. They make it very easy and efficient to gather trichomes or resin that would otherwise be lost. A handful of manufacturers make trim containers, or you can create your own.

vascular system   A plant's vascular system moves water, nutrients, minerals, and other substances throughout the tissues of the plant. It works much like the human circulatory system.

vegetative growth   The stage of growth after the seedling stage, in which cannabis plants grow vigorously and increase in size. They remain in the vegetative stage until the length of daylight decreases naturally in late summer or the grower reduces the amount of daylight that they receive to 12 hours over a 24-hour period.

wet trim   A type of trimming that involves removing all the leaves from the flowers when the cannabis is fresh and green. This is done just after harvest. Although it may be easier to trim these leaves before drying, most growers agree that it produces an inferior final product compared to cannabis that has been dry trimmed.

< BOTANICAL NAMES OF PLANTS IN THIS BOOK >

Botanical names list the genus and species of a plant. Because there are often many plants with the same common name, it can be helpful to know the botanical name to be sure you are referencing the proper plant. When researching plants, always make sure that the common name matches up with its botanical name.

COMMON NAME	BOTANICAL NAME
Alfalfa	*Medicago sativa*
Borage	*Borago officinalis*
Broad beans (also known as fava beans)	*Vicia faba*
Buckwheat	*Fagopyrum esculentum*
Burdock	*Arctium lappa*
Calendula	*Calendula officinalis*
Cayenne pepper	*Capsicum annuum*
Chamomile	*Matricaria chamomilla*
Chickweed	*Stellaria media*
Chicory	*Cichorium intybus*
Chives	*Allium schoenoprasum*
Chrysanthemum	*Chrysanthemum* spp.
Clove	*Syzygium aromaticum*
Clover (red)	*Trifolium pratense*
Clover (white)	*Trifolium repens*
Comfrey	*Symphytum officinale*
Coriander	*Coriandrum sativum*
Cowpeas	*Vigna unguiculata*
Curley dock	*Rumex crispus*
Daikon radish	*Raphanus sativus var. Longipinnatus*
Dandelion	*Taraxacum officinale*
Dill	*Anethum graveolens*
Eastern hemlock	*Tsuga canadensis*
Echinacea	*Echinacea purpurea, E. angustifolia*
Elecampane	*Inula helenium*
Eucalyptus	*Eucalyptus globulus*
Feverfew	*Tanacetum parthenium*
Field peas	*Pisum sativum*

COMMON NAME	BOTANICAL NAME
Fir	*Abies* spp.
Garlic mustard	*Alliaria petiolata*
Hairy vetch	*Vicia villosa*
Horsetail	*Equisetum arvense, Equisetum* spp.
Jerusalem artichoke	*Helianthus tuberosus*
Lambsquarters	*Chenopodium album*
Lemon balm	*Melissa officinalis*
Marshmallow	*Althaea officinalis*
Milk thistle	*Silybum marianum*
Mugwort	*Artemesia vulgaris*
Nasturtium	*Tropaeolum majus*
Oats	*Avena sativa*
Onions	*Allium cepa*
Oregano	*Origanum vulgare*
Peppermint	*Mentha piperita*
Pigweed	*Amaranthus* spp.
Pine	*Pinus* spp.
Red-rooted pigweed	*Amaranthus retroflexus*
Rosemary	*Salvia rosmarinus*
Sage	*Salvia officinalis, Salvia* spp.
Skullcap	*Scutellaria lateriflora*
Sorghum	*Sorghum bicolor*
Spruce	*Picea* spp.
Stinging nettle	*Urtica dioica*
Strawflower	*Xerochrysum bracteatum*
Sumac	*Rhus* spp.
Sunflower	*Helianthus annuus*
Sweet alyssum	*Lobularia maritima*
Tansy	*Tanacetum vulgare*
Thyme	*Thymus vulgaris*
Tobacco	*Nicotiana tabacum, Nicotiana* spp.
Tulsi (also called holy basil)	*Ocimum tenuiflorum*
Valerian	*Valeriana officinalis*
Wild grape	*Vitis* spp.
Willow tree	*Salix* spp.
Winter rye	*Lolium perenne*
Wormwood	*Artemisia absinthium*
Yarrow	*Achillea millefolium*

< ACKNOWLEDGMENTS >

I would like to start by thanking my wife, Bobbi. She supported me throughout the writing process and looked after our health, children, farm, and all the things that go into raising a family and taking care of the land, while I was busy working on this book. Without her, our family would not have been so well taken care of, especially during the coronavirus pandemic. Thank you, babe. I love you. Words could never fully express my love and appreciation for all you have done for our family.

I also want to thank the spirit and essence of the cannabis plant. This master plant has brought so much into my life, and I will always be indebted to it for all that it has given me. I will continue to educate and encourage people to form a relationship with her as she never ceases to amaze me. She possesses such wisdom and healing and is always willing to share this medicine with humans when we approach her with the love and respect that she deserves. I am committed to helping people nurture their own relationship with this sacred plant.

To the team of people at Sterling Publishing, I wish to thank everyone who had a hand in putting this book together: Renee Yewdaev, Jo Obarowski, Igor Satanovsky, Gavin Motnyk, and Linda Liang. And special thanks to my editor, Elysia Liang, who guided me through the writing process and kept both the writing and myself on track. Thanks also goes out to my friend and colleague Pat Crocker for recommending me for this project. It was this initial push that led to the creation of this book.

I would also like to thank the people who introduced me to cannabis in my teenage years and inspired me to learn to grow this plant. You know who you are. Those years were pivotal in the beginning of my journey. To all the old timers, growers, and breeders who kept working under the shadow of prohibition and under the threat of the law and criminal charges, you are the true OGs and legacy producers. You held on to the passion and desire to breed, produce, and provide this medicine to the people who sought it out and needed it the most. It is my hope that your work will be honored and that you will find a place for yourself in this new world of legalization.

As we move forward and the stigma surrounding cannabis fades away, I hope and pray that people will embrace this plant as the healer and sacred medicinal herb that she is. May the essence and beauty of this plant not get lost in the rushing green tide of corporate greed that has infiltrated the cannabis community. May the light of the cannabis plant shine brightly on all those who seek her with a pure heart, and may we reciprocate by sharing our love and passion for this blessed herb.

Lastly, I would like to express my gratitude for the Great Mystery of Life, for the unseen and eternal forces that move through our lives each and every day. And to the raw beauty and power of the natural world, thank you for serving as a constant reminder to be the best that I can be. It is this source of light and love that will truly move us all toward a regenerative future.

< BIBLIOGRAPHY >

Backes, Michael. *Cannabis Pharmacy: The Practical Guide to Medical Marijuana*. New York: Black Dog & Leventhal, 2014.

BD Editors. "Cultivar." Biology Dictionary. Last modified May 20, 2018. Accessed October 22, 2020. https://biologydictionary.net/cultivar/.

Cervantes, Jorge. *Marijuana Horticulture: The Indoor/Outdoor Medical Grower's Bible*. Vancouver, WA: Van Patten Publishing, 2006.

"Choosing the Best Cover Crops for Your Organic No-Till Vegetable System." Rodale Institute. Accessed October 30, 2020. https://rodaleinstitute.org/science/articles/choosing-the-best-cover-crops-for-your-organic-no-till-vegetable-system/.

Clarke, Robert Connell. *Marijuana Botany: An Advanced Study—The Propagation and Breeding of Distinctive Cannabis*. Oakland, CA: Ronin Publishing, 1981.

Clarke, Robert Connell, and Mark D. Merlin. *Cannabis: Evolution and Ethnobotany*. Berkeley and Los Angeles: University of California Press, 2013.

"Closed Loop Systems." DEM Pure Farms. Accessed October 28, 2020. http://dempurefarms.com/closed-loop-practices/.

Green, Greg. *The Cannabis Grow Bible: The Definitive Guide to Growing Marijuana for Recreational and Medical Use*, 3rd ed. Toronto: Green Candy Press, 2017.

Hillig, Karl. "Genetic Evidence for Speciation in Cannabis (*Cannabaceae*)." *Genetic Resources and Crop Evolution* 52, no. 2 (January 2005): 161–180. https://www.researchgate.net/publication/226862901_Genetic_Evidence_for_Speciation_in_Cannabis_Cannabaceae.

——. "A Systematic Investigation of Cannabis," PhD diss. Indiana University, 2005. https://www.researchgate.net/publication/281848590_A_Systematic_Investigation_of_Cannabis.

"Korean Natural Farming Inputs." Chris Trump Natural Farming. Accessed October 30, 2020. https://christrump.com/inputs/.

Lee, Martin A. *Smoke Signals: A Social History of Marijuana*. New York: Scribner, 2012.

Lewis, Mark A., Ethan B. Russo, and Kevin M. Smith. "Pharmacological Foundations of Cannabis Chemovars." *Planta Medica* 48, no. 4 (March 2018): 225–233. https://www.ncbi.nlm.nih.gov/pubmed/29161743.

Lowenfels, Jeff. *Teaming with Nutrients: The Organic Gardener's Guide to Optimizing Plant Nutrition*. Portland, OR: Timber Press, 2013.

——. *Teaming with Fungi: The Organic Gardener's Guide to Mycorrhizae*. Portland, OR: Timber Press, 2017.

Lowenfels, Jeff, and Wayne Lewis. *Teaming with Microbes: The Organic Gardener's Guide to the Soil Food Web*, rev. ed. Portland, OR: Timber Press, 2010.

Pavlis, Robert. *Soil Science for Gardeners: Working with Nature to Build Soil Health*. Gabriola Island, BC: New Society Publishers, 2020.

Rätsch, Christian. *Marijuana Medicine: A World Tour of the Healing and Visionary Powers of Cannabis*. Rochester, VT: Healing Arts Press, 1998.

"Regenerative Sun Grown Practices." Regenerative Cannabis Farming. Accessed October 30, 2020. https://regenerativecannabisfarming.org/practices.

The Rev. *True Living Organics: The Ultimate Guide to Growing All-Natural Marijuana Indoors*. Toronto: Green Candy Press, 2016.

Rosenthal, Ed. *Marijuana Pest and Disease Control: How to Protect Your Plants and Win Back Your Garden*. Oakland, CA: Quick American Archives, 2012.

Roy-Bolduc, Alice, and Mohamed Hijri. "The Use of Mycorrhizae to Enhance Phosphorus Uptake: A Way Out the Phosphorus Crisis." *Journal of Biofertilizers and Biopesticides* 2, no. 1 (July 2011). https://www.longdom.org/open-access/the-use-of-mycorrhizae-to-enhance-phosphorus-uptake-a-way-out-the-phosphorus-crisis-2155-6202.1000104.pdf.

Russo, Ethan B. "The Case for the Entourage Effect and Conventional Breeding of Clinical Cannabis: No 'Strain,' No Gain." *Frontiers in Plant Science* 9 (January 2019): 1969. https://pubmed.ncbi.nlm.nih.gov/30687364/.

Sulak, Dustin. "Cannabis Education." Healer. Accessed October 30, 2020. https://healer.com/cannabiseducation/.

Virginia Tech. "A Billion Years of Coexistence between Plants and Fungi." ScienceDaily (February 6, 2019). Accessed October 30, 2020. https://www.sciencedaily.com/releases/2019/02/190206123749.htm.

< RESOURCES >

CANNABIS SEED COMPANIES

NOTE: Since selling cannabis seeds can fall in a gray area depending on your local laws, most seed companies sell seeds as "souvenirs," "novelties," or "collectibles." No matter where you live, it is important to do your research and know the laws regulating the sale and purchase of cannabis seeds in your area.

Artizen Seed Shop
artizenseedshop.com

Heavily Connected Seed Bank
heavilyconnected.com

Hemp Depot
hempdepot.ca

Jordan of the Islands
jordanoftheislands.ca

Neptune Seed Bank
neptuneseedbank.com

Quebec Cannabis Seeds
quebeccannabisseeds.com

Regenerative Seed Company
regenerativeseeds.com

Staefli Farms
staefli.com

Xotic Seeds
xoticseeds.com

CANNABIS GROWING EQUIPMENT

Canada

Grow Buds
wegrowbuds.ca

Grow Daddy
growdaddycanada.com

The Grow Depot
thegrowdepot.ca

Indoor Growing Canada
indoorgrowingcanada.com

United States

Grow Buds
wegrowbuds.co

HTG Supply
htgsupply.com

Hydrobuilder
hydrobuilder.com

Saratoga Organics and Hydroponic Supply
saratogaorganics.com

GARDENING TOOLS AND EQUIPMENT

Gardener's Supply Company
gardeners.com

Johnny's Selected Seeds
johnnyseeds.com

Lee Valley Tools
leevalley.com/en-us

INSECTARIES

Applied Bio-nomics
appliedbio-nomics.com

Beneficial Insectary
insectary.com

BioBest
biobestgroup.com

Bio Works Inc.
bioworksinc.com

Koppert Biological Systems
koppert.com

SOIL MIXES AND SOIL AMENDMENTS

Black Swallow Living Soils
blackswallowsoil.com

BuildASoil, LLC
buildasoil.com

Dragonfly Earth Medicine
dragonflyearthmedicine.com

Kis Organics
kisorganics.com

The Soil King
thesoilking.com

Stepwell Soil Inc.
stepwellsoil.com

REGENERATIVE FARMING RESOURCES

Chris Trump Natural Farming
christrump.com

Dem Pure Farms
dempurefarms.com

Dr. Elaine's Soil Food Web
soilfoodweb.com

Regenerative Cannabis Farming
regenerativecannabisfarming.org

Rodale Institute
rodaleinstitute.org

The Science of Regenerative Organic

Cannabis Cultivation Conference
regenerativeorganiccannabis.com

Sun + Earth Certified
sunandearth.org

CANNABIS INFORMATION RESOURCES

Government of Canada
canada.ca/en/health-canada
/services/drugs-medication
/cannabis.html

Leafly
leafly.com
leafly.ca

OrganiGrow Canada
organigrowcanada.com

Seedfinder
en.seedfinder.eu

Strainly
strainly.io

United States Food and Drug Administration
https://www.fda.gov/news-events
/public-health-focus/fda
-regulation-cannabis-and
-cannabis-derived-products
-including-cannabidiol-cbd

Weedmaps
weedmaps.com

< FURTHER READING >

Appelhof, Mary, and Joanne Olszewski. *Worms Eat My Garbage: How to Set Up and Maintain a Worm Composting System*, 35th Anniversary Ed. North Adams, MA: Storey Publishing, 2017.

Backes, Michael. *Cannabis Pharmacy: The Practical Guide to Medical Marijuana*. New York: Black Dog & Leventhal, 2014.

Cervantes, Jorge. *Marijuana Horticulture: The Indoor/Outdoor Medical Grower's Bible*. Vancouver, WA: Van Patten Publishing, 2006.

Cho, Youngsang. *JADAM Organic Farming: The Way to Ultra-Low-Cost Agriculture*. Korea: JADAM, 2012.

Clarke, Robert Connell. *Marijuana Botany: An Advanced Study: The Propagation and Breeding of Distinctive Cannabis*. Oakland CA: Ronin Publishing, 1981.

Clarke, Robert Connell, and Mark D. Merlin. *Cannabis: Evolution and Ethnobotany*. Berkeley and Los Angeles: University of California Press, 2013.

Fukuoka, Masanobu. *The One-Straw Revolution: An Introduction to Natural Farming*. New York: New York Review of Books Classics, 2005.

Green, Greg. *The Cannabis Grow Bible: The Definitive Guide to Growing Marijuana for Recreational and Medical Use*, 3rd ed. Toronto: Green Candy Press, 2017.

Johnson, Jacob, and Karla Avila. *The Flowerdaze Farm Regenerative Guide to Cannabis: A Season-Long Recipe Book for the Beyond-Organic Gardener*. Toronto: BookBaby, 2020.

Lowenfels, Jeff. *Teaming with Fungi: The Organic Gardener's Guide to Mycorrhizae*. Portland, OR: Timber Press, 2017.

———. *Teaming with Nutrients: The Organic Gardener's Guide to Optimizing Plant Nutrition.* Portland, OR: Timber Press, 2013.

Lowenfels, Jeff, and Wayne Lewis. *Teaming with Microbes: The Organic Gardener's Guide to the Soil Food Web, Revised Edition.* Portland, OR: Timber Press, 2010.

Newcomb, Lawrence. *Newcomb's Wildflower Guide.* New York: Little, Brown and Company, 1989.

Phillips, Michael. *Mycorrhizal Planet: How Symbiotic Fungi Work with Roots to Support Plant Health and Build Soil Fertility.* White River Junction, VT: Chelsea Green Publishing, 2017.

Reddy, Rohini. *Cho's Global Natural Farming.* Bengaluru: South Asia Rural Reconstruction Association, 2011. ilcasia.files.wordpress. com/2012/02/chos-global-natural-farming-sarra.pdf.

Rosenthal, Ed. *Marijuana Grower's Handbook: Your Complete Guide for Medical and Personal Marijuana.* Oakland, CA: Quick American Publishing, 2010.

———. *Marijuana Pest and Disease Control: How to Protect Your Plants and Win Back Your Garden.* Oakland, CA: Quick American Archives, 2012.

Stamets, Paul. *Mycelium Running: How Mushrooms Can Help Save the World.* Berkeley, CA: Ten Speed Press, 2005.

Sweet, Tammi. *The Wholistic Healing Guide to Cannabis: Understanding the Endocannabinoid System, Addressing Specific Ailments and Conditions, and Making Cannabis-Based Remedies.* North Adams, MA: Storey Publishing, 2020.

< PICTURE CREDITS >

< INDEX >

Note: Page numbers in *italics* indicate mixes/recipes.

< ABOUT THE AUTHOR >

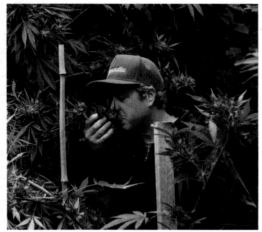

CREDIT: KIM SMITH

Alexis Burnett is an herbalist, farmer, and nature connection mentor who lives on traditional land of the Three Fires Confederacy and home of the Anishinabek Nation, also called Grey County, Ontario, Canada. He has been working with plants since childhood and has spent the last twenty-five years honing his craft as an herbalist and herb farmer. He lives with his wife and two kids on Rebel Roots Herb Farm (rebelrootsherbfarm.com), where they grow, sell, and ethically wildcraft more than fifty medicinal plants using organic and regenerative farming practices and produce high-quality herbal medicines. Rebel Roots is a DEM Pure certified farm and is committed to caretaking the land and building healthy communities in both the natural and human world. Their farm is home to Earth Tracks Outdoor School (earthtracks.ca), which connects people to nature and helps them cultivate a deep relationship with the Earth through courses and apprenticeship programs. These experiences cover such topics as foraging, community herbalism, naturalist training, wildlife tracking, bird language, and bush craft skills. Alexis is also one of the founders of the Heartwood Gathering (heartwoodgathering.ca), an annual three-day celebration of plants that takes place each summer in Ontario.

After the legalization of cannabis in Canada, Alexis founded OrganiGrow Canada. OrganiGrow Canada specializes in providing high-quality cannabis education backed by true experience, through online and in-person workshops. The Cannabis Home Growers course guides participants through the growing season from seed to harvest and shares extensive detail about every step of the process. Focusing specifically on "beyond" organic, regenerative growing practices, it includes dozens of hours of video, handouts, an online forum to ask questions, and live online meetings. The Cannabis Medicine Making Course teaches you to make cannabis-based medicinal products, such as salves, edibles, tinctures, oils, capsules, and more, at home from an herbalist's perspective. It covers how to properly calculate dosage and includes lessons on the endocannabinoid system, cannabinoids, terpenes, the therapeutic uses of cannabis medicine, and more. Both of these courses are offered online and are open to students from across the globe. To learn more about OrganiGrow Canada, visit organigrowcanada.com.